Year of the Onion

A Healing Journey <u>with</u> Cancer

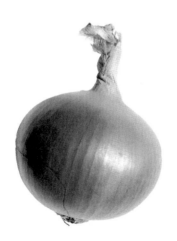

Deliah,

I so appreciate
all the musical
delight you have
brought into
my life!

Kathleen ♡

Year of the Onion

A Healing Journey <u>with</u> Cancer

"Out of the blue, an ordinary onion appeared
announcing the arrival of an extraordinary
experience that changed my life."

Kathleen Millat Johnson

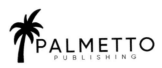

Charleston, SC
www.PalmettoPublishing.com

Year of the Onion: A Healing Journey <u>with</u> Cancer

First Edition

Editor: Shanen Johnson
Cover Design and Photography: Shanen Johnson
Paperback ISBN: 978-1-63837-749-8
eBook ISBN: 978-1-63837-750-4

The names of the doctors have been changed
for their privacy. Legal considerations prevent
the author from recommending any of the procedures
or products mentioned in the *Year of the Onion:
A Healing Journey <u>with</u> Cancer.*

I dedicate the *Year of the Onion: A Healing Journey <u>with</u> Cancer* to those who have the courage to examine their lives. I hope that you will find in it a valuable piece of information, an inspiring story and new ideas to explore as you follow my journey. Most of all, I offer this book as a way to say you are not alone.

"We must learn to reawaken and keep ourselves awake, not by mechanical aids, but by an infinite expectation of the dawn, which does not forsake us in our soundest sleep."

Henry David Thoreau

CONTENTS

Prologue.. xiii

Introduction xvii

Part One

1. In the Beginning... 3
2. The Search is On 12
3. I have *CUPS* 16
4. The Many Faces of Cancer...................................... 22
5. Spirit Matters... 27
6. Diving Deeper.. 32
7. Who to Tell? What to Tell? When to Tell? 42
8. Green Medicine 48
9. Psychics and a Haunting Dream 57
10. Eureka! 61
11. Now is the Hour.. 67
12. The Other Shoe Drops 72
13. "Heck No" to Chemo... 78
14. The Waiting Room 82
15. Survivors and Supporters.. 87

Part Two

16. What's Going on Down There?.............................. 95
17. Searching for Answers 101
18. What Now? 104

Part Three

19. The Boogie Man Under the Bed............................ 115
20. Together Again... 129
21. Standing in the Paradox... 135

Part Four

22. Meditation... 143

23. The Wisdom of Dreams... 155

24. Intuition and Guidance 181

25. A "Whole Brain" Approach to Making Decisions............ 198

26. Questions to Ask Your Doctor 204

27. Recommended Books... 209

Acknowledgements 219

Author's Biography 221

PROLOGUE

Beautiful South Carolina, a place I have called home for the past twenty years, with its brown sugar beaches, meandering rivers and tidal creeks, shrimp boats, cruise ships, gardens brimming over with gardenias and camellias, rainbow-colored mansions, cobblestone streets... I could go on and on about what makes Charleston unique and often listed as the number one tourist destination in the world.

Coming from gray Ohio, where deer, squirrels, rabbits and raccoons make up much of the wildlife, I was fascinated to find this sub-tropical state teeming with exotic creatures like alligators, armadillos, pelicans, dolphins, sea turtles, anoles and... unfortunately giant cockroaches and fire ants!

Charleston also teems with tourists (looking *not* so exotic) in their oversized t-shirts and Bermuda shorts wandering around downtown relishing local seafood, sampling pralines, grits, pulled pork, fried okra and other southern fare. Around every corner, tours are offered with themes of the Civil War, Gullah Culture, Plantations and Gardens, Pirates, Churches and Ghosts. There is so much to explore in Charleston that a bronze plaque on one downtown building jokes, "Nothing of historical significance happened on this corner."

I have my own favorite spots in Charleston and they cost nothing to enjoy. Driving out of Charleston toward the nearby town of Summerville, there is a road I love to take to visit my daughter and grandson—a scenic highway with gigantic live oak trees that border the road for about ten miles. State Route 61 (also known as Ashley River Road) is a two-lane highway that was once a dirt carriage lane to three famous plantations: Drayton Hall, Magnolia Gardens and Plantation and Middleton Place, all thriving in the late 1700's and 1800's. They are now popular tourist attractions still busy hosting visitors from around the world.

I call it a little piece of heaven, as all signs of commerce disappear, and I enter a natural tunnel of glittering green and gold, sunlight and shadow. Looking up, I can see the tips of the tree branches meeting overhead of the highway. I feel as if I am entering a cathedral; the sense of the sacred is so strong that I often ask any passengers with me to hold their thoughts for a few minutes so we can soak up the natural beauty in silence.

Sunlight, as strong as a strobe light, bounces across my windshield and nearly blinds me. I have to put on my sunglasses, then take them off just as suddenly when the road darkens into patches of inky black shadows. The play of dark and light can be distracting, especially when you are trying to stay alert for any deer that might dart out from the woods or a meandering armadillo whose escape ploy is to jump three feet up in the air right in line with your front bumper!

Live oak trees stand like giants; their limbs reaching out almost touching my car. They have a sensuous presence and hold the history of the South, both beautiful and terrible, in their branches. I miss them more than the ocean when I leave home. These are trees that open wide and hug you back.

The sunlit opening at the end of the tree tunnel gradually becomes larger and brighter. Then, whoosh... I am ejected into an ordinary world of flat grassy fields, small rural homes and a road sign pointing the way to Summerville, South Carolina.

I straighten up in my driver's seat, aware I will soon be taking an abrupt right turn; it's a shortcut that will eliminate the wait at the next intersection's traffic light. I click on my turn signal and begin to slow down, relishing the last of my green meditation. I feel lucky to be alive and living in such a gloriously diverse environment. Those ten miles of nature's blessing are just what I needed for my peace of mind. "Just another day in paradise," I say out loud to myself. I am unaware that in another minute my life will change drastically; the year of the onion is about to begin.

INTRODUCTION

This is a story of having cancer, searching for the source, getting treatment and surviving cancer. It involves a cat, a dog, an onion, a death, dreams, therapy and surrender. My cancer appeared in 2018, continued through 2019 and I was "all clear" in 2020. As we enter 2021, I continue to be well.

Writing this book has been a way to digest the experiences that cancer presented to me. My journey helped me answer the questions of what happened in my past and why cancer came into my life. I want to share what I've learned from the physical, mental, emotional and spiritual aspects of my journey, hoping my experiences will be meaningful to readers and be an example of one way to approach a cancer diagnosis. I chose the "middle path" between the medical view and my inner guidance.

It took six months, many visits to specialists and two trips to the Mayo Clinic for physicians to solve the mystery of where my cancer originated. As the medical team put together the puzzle pieces, I was on a search of my own. My inner detective work indicated that the probable location where the cancer could be hiding, ticking away like a time bomb, was a site in my body that held memories, shame and vulnerability.

People ask me how I beat cancer. "I didn't try to 'beat' anything," I answer. I followed a path of understanding cancer, as it was revealed to me, step by step and day by day. I sought peace and acceptance through inner work and sometimes I just staggered along in the dark, terrified. I researched and educated myself regarding the medical model, explored my past, read inspiring books and kept an open mind, trying everything from canned asparagus to psychic readings. I listened to my dreams, worked with symbols as messengers and paid attention to my intuition. I respected my doctors and the medical models presented to me and I trusted my ability to make my own decisions.

I call this book *a healing journey _with_ cancer* because I was learning about myself as I walked with cancer, peeling layers of my past away. I stayed awake and aware of all the things that were happening around and within me. I operated from a belief that the whole world was talking to me through my conscious and unconscious mind.

This is not a book about a cancer cure, although I mention a few treatments that I learned about along the way. (Disclaimer: I am sharing them—not recommending them.) My story is about how I listened to my body, mind and soul, and let cancer "talk" to me.

I make no claim that this way of healing is for everybody. Each one of us has an opportunity to choose what cancer means to us and how it affects our life. Everyone's journey is different, heading to destinations unknown, but one constant remains; once you have cancer, you are never the same.

Part One

CHAPTER 1

In the Beginning

Wheeee! No one else is on the shortcut, so I take the curves of the road fast, relishing the swing and sway of my car. After three curves, the serpentine road straightens out just in time for a quick stop before intersecting the highway. I stop at the stop sign, check for traffic and pull out onto the main road. Pushing on the gas pedal, I get a surprise—no get up and go! I press down on the gas pedal again and still my car won't accelerate beyond 15mph. *Damn! It's always something with cars,* I think, *but surely my car is too new to be having any big problems.* I pull over to the side of the road and consider the facts: I have a towing service, no one has rear-ended me, it's daytime and there's a filling station in sight. I tell myself to take a breath and calm down.

I look around the floor mat at my feet—nothing amiss, so I explore under the brake and gas pedals with my fingers. The brake pedal is clear, but something that I can't see has blocked the gas pedal. I give it a hard tug and out pops a yellow onion about the size of a tennis ball!

Where did this onion come from and how did it roll to this exact spot to halt my car? I could only deduce that it came from the back seat and rolled under my front seat, landing under the pedal. But I never put my groceries in the front or back seats, always in the trunk of my car in a big plastic container. I sit in my car holding the culprit in my hands, wondering, *how did this onion get there?*

I've lost things in my car before and know from looking under the seats that there's a tangled mess under there. A jumble of wires, springs and seat adjustment tracks leave open just one small area about 4-5 inches wide. One narrow lane goes straight through the middle of all that gadgetry and somehow the swing and sway of the curves of the road impelled this mysterious onion to roll from the back to the front of the car through that limited space. And just like a billiard ball seeking a pocket, that onion found a resting place under my gas pedal. Unbelievable!

Removing the onion solved the acceleration problem and I proceeded to drive unhampered to my daughter's home a few miles away. I told her the funny story when I arrived and showed her the problem onion. "Any idea how this got under my gas pedal?" I asked her. No answers from her or from other people I would later ask. I continued thinking about this incident for a few days, dissecting it as if it were a dream, looking at objects (onion, gas pedal, car), settings (daytime, sunshine, easy drive), dynamics (driving, blocked energy source, obstruction), and emotions (confusion, anger, relief). Here's how I put together the scenario:

I am on the road (of life) in my car (body) taking a trip (out of my neighborhood). I am in the driver's seat (seemingly in control) and I take the curves of the road fast for fun (risks), when an object (round, organic) blocks my forward motion (life force) and I lose my power (movement) and get stuck. The problem comes from the back of my car (subconscious) to the front (consciousness) and renders my forward movement (energy) stalled.

What should I do with this information? Avoid wayward onions or shortcuts? It wasn't clear to me at that time why my car's progress was impaired. I was just doing what I often do, driving to see my daughter and grandson. I stored this strange incident away in my mind for later contemplation. I would have to wait until something more would be revealed—and I didn't have to wait too long.

A few months later in mid-September, I was lying in bed one morning doing my usual wake-up routine of stretching, deep breathing, tensing and relaxing my body. It is something I have been doing for decades and it energizes me for the day ahead. (Recently, I found there is a word for it—*pandiculation*.) As I was slowly twisting, turning, tensing and releasing, my right hand skimmed over something as hard and round as an *onion* in my right groin! A cold trickle of fear ran through me as I touched it again and there it was—a lump as big as a hen's egg. *How did it get there? Don't panic and do your usual catastrophic thinking,* I cautioned myself, *not all lumps are cancer.*

But of course I panicked! I watched the clock until it

read 8:00 a.m. and then called my doctor's office asking for an appointment as soon as possible. "Yes, I can come in today," I told them, thinking right this minute would not be too soon for me!

Forty-five minutes later I was at the primary care office being told that my regular doctor, Dr. McMurray, had not come to work that day due to a problem with her pregnancy. Would it be okay with me if the physician's assistant saw me? "Sure, that's fine," I affirmed, just wanting someone who would tell me everything was all right.

It was a little disconcerting when a young blonde woman named Meghan came into the exam room and introduced herself as the physician's assistant. I told myself not to worry—get used to medical personnel looking 18 years old! Pretty Meghan could have been a cover model for a surfer's magazine, except she was wearing a white lab coat.

"Oh, that's just a lymph node," she explained, examining my groin area. "It's inflamed and swollen. It's doing its job of handling some infection. Have you been sick recently?" she asked.

"Not for a few months," I told her. "But I was terribly sick back in June. I was so ill for several weeks that I stayed in bed most of the time. I finally saw Dr. McMurray and she diagnosed it as a virus, saying there wasn't anything she could do for me but symptom relief." The virus was devastating and it came with a nasty eye infection, too. I kept drinking products with electrolytes since I felt like my entire electrical system had crashed. I complained to my daughter, "I'm so weak that even if the house were on fire, I wouldn't have the energy to get out of bed."

Later, I recalled that while I was so sick, I had had a disturbing dream of seeing parasites coming out of my body. I wrote it down and decided it must have been connected to the virus I was experiencing. It was a disgusting dream, but I felt that it was telling me something important because of my intense feeling of revulsion.

"See this chart?" Meghan pointed to one on the wall showing the systems in the body. The lymph system was outlined in long red "snakes" trailing up and down the arms, legs, neck, torso, running everywhere in the body. "No need to worry," she reassured me again. "It's just a swollen lymph node. Possibly from that virus. It'll return to normal."

As usual, I had panicked. I have always been a catastrophic thinker! *This was nothing,* I told myself, when I could exhale at last, *nothing but an inflamed lymph node.* At the reception desk in the hallway where I stood checking out, I exchanged a weak smile with the office staff, relieved it was something minor. But still, there was a nagging thought that I wished I had seen my regular doctor.

Soon enough however, I did see Dr. McMurray because in the following two weeks after seeing Meghan, my heart began to flutter, stop and start. I thought it might be my thyroid. Time for another test to see if I was on the right dosage of thyroid meds.

"I don't detect anything unusual," Dr. McMurray said, listening to my heart with her stethoscope. "If you would take your pulse when you have one of these episodes," she continued, "and count the beat for fifteen seconds, then multiply that by four, we could have more data."

"I never can find my pulse, much less do the math," I laughed. "I was thinking maybe the heart arrhythmia had something to do with my thyroid." I like to give Dr. McMurray my diagnosis and she is always a good sport about it.

As she looked up the dates of my last thyroid test, I reported, "Oh, by the way, I was just here two weeks ago when you were out sick. I saw Meghan. Her diagnosis was that I have an inflamed lymph node."

"Oh?" Dr. McMurray said, as she raised her eyebrows.

As I told the story of how surprisingly big and hard my lymph node was, Dr. McMurray's forehead furrowed as she asked in a no-nonsense voice, "Do you mind putting on a gown? I'd like to see it."

She examined my groin, pushing gently around on the lump, sensing how moveable it was. Her face appeared troubled.

"This is nothing to fool around with," she said, concerned. "I'm calling right now to schedule a scan for you."

That cold trickle of fear visited me again. *Oh God, this could be something after all!*

Things moved quickly; a scan was scheduled in a few days at the hospital, then in another week, another test, then a procedure to aspirate fluid from the lymph node. A few weeks later I was back in my doctor's office nervously waiting for the verdict. I had told no one except my daughter, stepdaughter and sweetheart that something was up with my health.

I surmised that by the way Dr. McMurray entered the exam room, I would know my fate. If she entered and walked forward, shutting the door behind her without turning around, it would be good news. If she entered and turned to face the door to close it with her back toward me, it meant bad news. I intuited that those few seconds she turned from me, she needed to compose herself.

Dr. McMurray entered the room and for a moment I thought she was walking straight towards me, but she stopped and turned around facing the door to close it. *Oh no...* My heart sank and I knew my life would be completely changed in a few moments.

Her next move nailed me in my coffin of fear as she pulled her chair closer to mine. I left my body and watched from above. This was the scene in my life's movie where I get bad news, the music swells, I cry, and then the next chapter begins—my life as a cancer patient.

But first came the information download, the details of the tests and reports on what had been done. Looking directly into my eyes, Dr. McMurray said the dreaded words, "It's cancer. I'm so sorry."

The lab results and surgeon's notes stated that the aspiration revealed squamous cancerous cells in my lymph node—stage three cancer.

"It is not like it used to be," she continued quickly. "There are treatments that work for cancer. I will be here on your team. You can call me anytime and I'll get back to you as soon as I can. You are not alone." Tears sprang to my eyes at her kindness and I was thankful she was so quick to act.

I did not believe this was happening to me. I never thought I would get cancer even though I had been with my mother through her cancer journey from 2011 to 2013 when she died. Her cancer was the result of taking hormonal supplements for thirty years. Her death from inflammatory breast cancer was a nightmare of two years of torture that no pain pill she took could alleviate. The memory of cancer ravenously eating away at her breasts and torso was still fresh in my mind as was the smell of rotting flesh in my nostrils. Her death was so long and brutal that I had been traumatized. I knew cancer, and I knew its power.

Numbly, I gathered my purse and the notes I wrote from Dr. McMurray's report and walked out of the office feeling like a robot. *How could this be happening?* A nurse, who had taken my vitals, came running out to the lobby to catch me leaving, having overheard the news already. She didn't say a word as she gave me a big hug, turned and ran back into the office. Now I realized I was marked with a big "C" on my forehead.

I didn't want to tell anyone that it was cancer—not yet, not even to alert my daughters, Shanen and Rochelle or my companion, Nick. Maybe, if I didn't say the C-word, it wouldn't be true. Trick or Treat night was coming and I had a big bag of candy bars in the cupboard waiting for me (I mean, the trick or treaters): miniature Butterfingers, Hershey bars, and Almond Joys. I reasoned that I needed them far more than the kids. I would drown my feelings not in drink, but by going into a sugar coma!

A few hours later found me finishing the whole big bag of candy, one gooey bar after another. I could eat candy guilt-free at last; no use worrying about getting fat or ruining my health with that devil sugar! I had cancer, so what the hell? Eat the chocolate! And I did. I savored the flavors, texture, and smells, chewing and chewing one candy bar after the next. Completely stuffed and surrounded by candy wrappers, I laid down on the couch feeling sick.

Dusk faded into night as I stretched out and watched the sky darken through the living room window. I lit a big candle on the coffee table to keep me company as I tried to wrap my mind around the enormity of the day's diagnosis. *I have cancer, I have cancer...* I kept saying to myself, and that lymph node was full of it. How could I not have known?

Then I remembered: *the onion*! It represented something jamming up my energy, slowing my car/journey down to a crawl. This is what that onion had been telling me. A wave of peace came over me when I realized that the strange symbolic scenario that stopped my car had been a forewarning of my body losing power. The location of the "jam" was also symbolic. The onion, almost the same size as my swollen lymph node, was located in a V-shaped angle where the gas pedal and the floor intersect, somewhat like the intersection of my leg and torso—my groin. Four months ago, this car incident had alerted me with that onion, warning me as to what was about to arrive uninvited into my life. I closed my eyes and prayed. If this is my path, so be it.

CHAPTER 2

The Search is On

Where was the original site of the cancer? That was the question the doctors needed to know in order to treat me. It was in my lymph node, filled with stage three squamous cell cancer, but it had to originate from some other place in my body; my rectum, anal area, ovaries, vagina, or from a melanoma hiding between my toes? Or could it be in my breasts, like my mother's cancer? "Would you mind taking an AIDS test?" the doctors asked, wanting to cover all the bases.

I finally ended up at a surgeon's office who informed me that the first thing to do was to get rid of that HUGE lymph node. All my doctors were fascinated by the size of it. Several meetings were held by my team of doctors shaking their heads in confusion; me and my lymph node with its unidentified primary cancer site were the medical curiosity of the month.

The surgery to remove the lymph node was a simple one, done as an out-patient at the hospital. The incision in my groin was only a few inches long and presented no pain at all. The lymph node was now gone, but the question continued to plague the doctors: where was the original site of the cancer? I was sent to a dermatologist, had a mammogram, a colonoscopy and a Pap smear. Nothing showed up. I was prodded and poked, my vagina stretched and scraped. I knelt on a stool at the end of an exam table to have my rectum examined several times, taking advantage of being on my knees to pray that this uncomfortable exam would be over quickly!

Several doctors on my team felt sure it was in the anal area because of the location of the lymph node. One doctor found some dysplasia cells in my vagina, which meant they were slightly off from normal, but not cancerous. The mystery continued to taunt the doctors.

With my doctors' approval, I decided to go to the Mayo Clinic in Jacksonville, Florida to see what they could find. Surely, at this state-of-the-art medical mecca, I could get some answers. Off I drove the six hours from Charleston, South Carolina to Florida hoping to get a diagnosis so I could move on to the next step.

The Mayo Clinic is an impressive medical center with lovely grounds, trees, ponds and walkways winding their way through grassy lawns. The red brick buildings are reassuringly solid with well-designed and nicely decorated interiors. It is here that they have advanced systems for treating patients, known throughout the world. I had a schedule of doctors to see in my hand and followed the instructions easily, amazed that there was no waiting anywhere for appointments.

Thankfully, I was not alone on this visit. I had contacted a good friend who lived in a town near Jacksonville and she had invited me to stay with her to avoid the extra cost of an overnight or two at a hotel. Not only did Worth provide shelter, but she accompanied me to my appointments at Mayo. She had the experience of having had cancer three times with no recurrence for thirty years. Her background as a nurse, lymphatic massage therapist and a Buddhist was a gift for keeping me calm while I wanted to freak out. She held my hand during some of the more painful exams and asked medical questions as my advocate. Everyone should be so lucky to have an angel like Worth by their side!

The Mayo Clinic, with their excellent doctors and latest technology, told me at the end of the day they did not have any answers for me. After an overnight visit with Worth, I left Florida and drove home to Charleston disappointed and still questioning. Where was the cancer's origin?

(Side note to the reader: My doctor's office in Charleston did not fax my records to them as they reassured me they would. The admitting doctor I saw at Mayo had to type in all my information, which took away valuable time from my appointment. Thankfully, I kept my notes, lab results, phone conversations and questions in a big manila envelope that I brought with me to Florida. I learned that even though I checked and rechecked, reminded and nearly harassed the Charleston doctor's office staff to fax my file on time to Mayo, this wasn't done even for my second visit to the Mayo Clinic. Keep your information with you at all times and bring it to all appointments. Write down notes regarding phone conversations, dates, times, doctors' names, lab reports, contact numbers and procedures done. You legally own your scans and test results and they will be released to you; however, there may be a form or two to fill out, a small charge and it may take a few days to have them released or faxed. If you want to pick them up in person, call ahead and find out where the medical records department is located. This will save you from wandering around the huge hospital maze. Being organized can eliminate so much stress; it's worth the time and care involved.)

I had nothing concrete to report to my Charleston medical team when I returned home. The mystery continued.

CHAPTER 3

I have *CUPS*

My research on the computer was giving me lots of possible locations, all equally horrifying: sinuses, mouth, brain, liver, adrenals, appendix, skin, follicles, bones. Wherever there were cells, there could be cancer. For the time being, I was diagnosed as having *CUPS*—an acronym meaning *Cancer of Unknown Primary Site.*

My daughter, Shanen, was helping me research information over the internet to see what we could find; looking for a new discovery, a future clinical trial that looked promising, the latest medications and alternative options. Radiation and chemotherapy were still coming up as the most common treatments for cancer. They have had top billing for the past sixty years. All that money, all that research, all the deaths and suffering of millions of people and sadly, that was the best we had to use against cancer.

Maybe if chemotherapy and radiation didn't kill you, maybe if you could stand the effects of poisoning your body with toxic chemicals, then maybe, just maybe, you might survive cancer. It was my fantasy that a surgeon would cut it out and I could be done with the whole thing. I tried to remember the reassuring words of Dr. McMurray: "Cancer's not a death sentence anymore."

My daughter and I continued our research, looking up cancer diets, herbal cures, fasting, Macrobiotics, raw foods, vitamins, supplements, coffee colonics, apricot pits, celery juice... The information we found on the subject was vast. Miso soup and mushroom supplements were two recommendations she made based on radiation poisoning studies, along with ginger and turmeric for pain and inflammation. Shanen, trained as an Integrative Health Coach, went over all my vitamins, honing in on what she believed were the most helpful and repeatedly begged, "Mom, drink more water!"

We also ordered a case of canned asparagus to try, since a friend's husband with cancer was trying this cure and believed it was helping. As for asparagus, I love it fresh and steamed, but canned is a different animal— soggy, brown and disgusting! I tried, I really did, to eat the murky mush, but gave up. I did enjoy the fresh organic vegetable and fruit juice that my daughter often made me from a blend of apples, carrots, lemons and celery. There is nothing like fresh juice and better yet, to have someone make it for you!

She knew my love of sweets and admonished me to stay away from sugar. I admit it, I am addicted to sugar. All the health sites and health gurus proclaim that cancer cells love sugar, too. I knew I had to stop eating it! I tried to be good, but I had to have a Pepsi once in a while. When I asked a doctor about eating sugar, he said go ahead and have that cookie! (He didn't know that one cookie was just the beginning for an addict like me.) He continued, adding: "The only proof we have of a direct connection between what we put in our mouths to cancer is tobacco."

However, there is another view of cancer that says food plays a big part in causing it and curing it. Many studies show diet is very important, as well as keeping the colon clean through the use of coffee enemas or colonics, which is highly recommended for most cancer patients. Some health experts say that cancer cannot exist in an alkaline environment. A friend of mine with cancer took this advice to heart and squeezed lemons on everything she ate or drank but, sadly to say, it didn't work for her.

My mom, a health food consultant with forty years of experience working in health food stores and studying nutrition, believed that a correct diet and supplements could cure anything. She tried to heal herself of stage four invasive inflammatory breast cancer with eighty vitamins a day. Yes, that's eighty! After a couple years of suffering, she lamented that she should have had her breasts cut off in the beginning when the sores began to appear.

I believe surgery would have been easier on her and maybe it could have saved her life. She lived to be eighty-nine years old (cancer occurred at age 86). Ironically, Mom had helped many people with health problems throughout her years in the natural health field, but in the end, her vast knowledge of health and nutrition did not save her. I will say that living to be 89 years old is a testament for vitamins, supplements and the many alternative therapies she tried. She died with beautiful skin, good circulation, a clear mind and was walking up and down nine flights of steps at her apartment building every day, until cancer caught up to her.

I watched my mother fight cancer for three years while she tried everything from visualization, contacting her guardian angels, taking *Essiac Tea* (a well-known natural herbal cancer tonic found at health food stores), prayer and vitamin therapy. Friends laid healing hands on her, gave her massages and reiki treatments, meditated and prayed with her. In retrospect, I think she truly believed she would beat cancer and then perhaps write a book about it since she was quite a good writer. Thinking ahead to illustrate her book, she had a friend take photos of her breasts every month to monitor the progress she hoped she was making.

After six months of looking at the grisly photos, Mom finally realized that she was not gaining any ground with all her alternative techniques. Her breasts continued to deteriorate. She cancelled the photo sessions and came to terms with the fact that even with her lifetime of health wisdom, she had been outwitted by cancer. Because her prayers were not answered, she lost her faith in God and lost her life in the spring of 2013.

Why hadn't she considered surgery in the first place? Mom had been at odds with medical doctors since her youth, when she believed some renegade nurse or crazy doctor tried to poison her while she was in the hospital recuperating from a urinary tract infection. "I think it was arsenic poisoning," she always said when she told the story, "because for years after, doctors said my urinary tract was so scarred, I must have been given some kind of acid." Whether this was true or just her conclusion, I never knew.

But I knew for a fact she had to take daily antibiotics for years to control the bacteria in her urinary tract, which she believed ruined her immune system, resulting in many bouts with illnesses throughout her life. This "arsenic poisoning" story was one of her many dramatic stories about bad doctors. It affected my attitude, too, as I grew up wary of doctors and medical systems.

Mom always said, if the time came when it was evident that she was not going to recover or would have to live in unrelenting pain, she would commit suicide. She had all the literature from the Hemlock Society about how to do it, too. But in the end, her fear was that if she bungled the job, she would live on with terrible complications and become a "vegetable"—a burden on her family. She decided not to take the chance.

I thought about suicide, if and how I would do it, and what help I would need to make sure it was done right. Could I ask my daughter or step-daughter to help me? "Here, honey, make sure this plastic bag stays sealed securely around my head and neck until I turn blue." What an abhorrent request!

I researched Mexican cancer clinics and wondered if I went to Mexico and their cures didn't work, could I hire someone there to kill me? And what if the person I hired took the money and ran before doing the deed? Or what if they didn't do it right? How does one go about arranging such a thing?

Wait a minute, forget Mexico! I realized that there are some states right here in the USA who have right-to-death laws with doctor-assisted suicides. Part of the criteria is having a doctor confirm you are within six months of dying. And this diagnosis must be renewed if you live beyond six months. You may have to establish a residency in that state, find a doctor there and wait and see how you decline—all of which involves time, money and help. Suicide is not always easy.

The more I read about cancer, the more ridiculous it appeared to try to outsmart it. It didn't seem to me that there was any sure way to *fight* cancer. And I knew I wasn't a fighter anyway. For some reason, I wanted to make peace with cancer. The "onion warning" kept me from panicking, because for me, it was assurance that this cancer experience, however it turned out, was predestined.

Living in limbo with the odd diagnosis of CUPS, was my destiny for now. The acronym for me stood for a Contradiction Undermining my Peace and Sanity.

CHAPTER 4

The Many Faces of Cancer

In my cancer research on the internet, I came upon a story of a young woman named Christina Baldwin. Lovely Christina had a huge viewer base because she was very smart, articulate and had a warm, natural way of talking to the viewers on a variety of subjects. I caught the end of a popular segment following Christina as she lost weight for her wedding day. She shared her diet struggles with her viewers until there she was—a trim beautiful bride marrying a handsome guy in a lovely fairy tale wedding.

Unfortunately, soon after their marriage, she received the diagnosis of breast cancer. For more than two years, she informed her viewing audience daily about her struggle, medical treatments and emotions as she fought for her life. Then came another surprise for Christina and her husband: an unplanned pregnancy and birth of a darling little girl.

I followed Christina on her roller coaster ride, as she detailed her cancer research, doctor visits, hopes and fears. After months, she finally gave up on the medical cures and began putting all her energy into eating a raw diet, the same one that had helped her lose weight for her wedding. She gave her fan base a daily report, all of us hoping the diet might work again. It didn't. Devastated, she decided to give up the raw food approach and go back to the chemo treatments as her doctor had advised. Much to her surprise, a chemotherapy drug started to reduce the size of her cancer. She regretted that she hadn't stuck it out with the original medical treatment—but how do we know if it would have worked?

I was tuning into her website almost daily. I had come to love Christina and her brave family: a steadfast mom, a supportive, loving husband and the beautiful little girl she had birthed right in the middle of her cancer journey. One day, there was a shock when I tuned in to see a resigned Christina and her downcast husband sitting on her bed as she looked directly into the camera and told us that her fight was over. It would be a matter of days, perhaps hours before she died, she sadly explained. She thanked us, her viewers, for our loyalty and prayers. A day later, I checked in on her site and found one of her friends, gently telling viewers that Christina had died. Christina, a young, beautiful newlywed and new mother had lost her life to breast cancer. She was one of 40,000 such women who die from breast cancer every year in the United States.

It struck me then that you can armor yourself with the latest cancer information, enlist thousands to pray for your healing, try the latest treatments, eat the perfect diet, enroll in clinical studies, go to the best doctors all over the world, and still die. You could be the most motivated person, courageous, able to afford the latest state-of-the-art treatments like superstar Farrah Fawcett with anal cancer—and still you can't count on healing. You might have children to raise, important duties to fulfill, a lifetime leading to a Nobel Peace Prize, but cancer doesn't care! Those rogue cells want to live as much as you do!

Still, I continued looking at sites that claimed to have cancer cures: herbs, diet, prayer, changing your personality, rewiring your brain, mindfulness and guided imagery. I took my vitamins, drank pure water and tried to eat healthfully except for a Pepsi or two a month. Immunotherapy was looking promising, laser light therapy was a possibility, new drugs were coming out monthly. Something should work! Look how far medical research has come with helping patients who can now live with HIV!

Currently, medical doctors advocate for surgery, radiation and chemotherapy for most cancers and give you a life expectancy by statistics. The statistics let you look at how many people lived and for how long and how many died, but they don't let you know how impacted and impaired those are who lived. One person's quality of life may not be acceptable to another.

Just when you despair, you hear a story of someone almost dying of cancer and then miraculously recovering to live a healthy life. Or the reverse: someone who takes great care with their diet, exercises, is full of energy and radiates health, suddenly has cancer and before you know it, is dead! Cancer plays with us like a cat with a mouse.

"Don't do any research on cancer," several of my doctors advised me. "The internet is full of misinformation and ads for potions and cures that are a waste of money. You'll end up scared and confused." But I kept at it, reading about Mexico's cancer clinics, researching M.D. Anderson Hospital, Cancer Cures of America, various health treatment centers and health spas that exist all over the world.

I talked by phone with a staff person from a famous Mexican clinic in Tijuana that advertised positive stories of cancer cures using laetrile, coffee enemas and nutrition. They dropped contact with me when I did not immediately sign up and fly down. I couldn't tell them what kind of cancer I had, since at that time I still did not know. I'm sure this sounded suspicious to them, as much as I was also suspicious of flying to a clinic, sight unseen, in Mexico.

I was trying to find a way to deal with cancer that felt right for me. I had decided I would not *battle* cancer even though it seemed to be my worst enemy. What if that were not completely true? What if there was something I needed to learn and cancer was my teacher? The medical model of "burn and destroy" did not inspire me with confidence and I wasn't sure if natural or alternative cures were for me either. Perhaps there was a middle path of blending the two.

That's when I found Doctor Low Dog's story online. An Indigenous woman, Dr. Tieraona Low Dog, began her career in medicine as an herbalist, midwife and natural healer, then went on to get a standard medical degree. I watched a video of her speaking at a conference on healing plants where she spotlighted Saw Palmetto as a superior herbal cure for prostate problems. I was very impressed with her. Later in my research, I found out that Dr. Low Dog (drlowdog.com) once had breast cancer and chose to walk the middle path of using both the natural alternatives and conventional medical treatments. It was a hard time for her, as she felt certain she was going to die. Much to her surprise, she didn't. She is cancer-free and you can view her cancer story on the internet. She did not choose one way of healing over the other; she integrated both the medical and natural health options. *Great*, I thought. *I, too, would walk the middle path.*

CHAPTER 5

Spirit Matters

For three years I watched my mom's tortuous decline, as cancer ate into her body, leaving it looking like the aftermath of a shark attack. I didn't think I had much of a chance as an older, overweight, under-exercised woman who ate sugar, dairy and all kinds of "bad" foods. I didn't drink much water and made fun of those who had to constantly "hydrate." Maybe that was the reason for my cancer. Or was it my moodiness, years of depression, negative thinking, unresolved issues, people-pleasing ways or my unforgiving nature? With all that, I certainly fit the cancer psychological profile!

Cancer compels one to look at death. It forced me to take account of my spiritual values and see what was there to support me. After years of study, I had settled on a patchwork mix of Taoism, Buddhism, Christ Consciousness and Native American beliefs. I realized that I still didn't know what Life was all about—except to be kind, surrender ego, and strive to be as peaceful and as loving a person as possible.

I am not a "born again" but a "go within." Now, with cancer nipping at my heels, maybe I should meditate more, rev up my kundalini, travel to South America and try that mind-blowing vine, ayahuasca. I was considering all options.

Actually, there was something practical I could do: make out my bucket list which included a cross country trip in an RV to visit New England in the fall or a river cruise through Europe with friends. Obviously, I needed to get my finances in order, update my will and examine my bank accounts and investments. I went through my personal belongings, boxed up and labeled treasured items to be given to special people in my life, wrote my obituary notice and pondered: *how much time did I have?*

I made a surreal trip to a funeral home to make my final plans. There, I found quite a vast commercial market that dead people provide for the living. I could get my fingerprint permanently pressed on a pendant or my ashes suspended in a glass sculpture. Gift items were displayed on shelves all around the funeral home: souvenirs of a life available for sale at a big price. I decided I wanted to be cremated with my ashes sent to Ohio and buried next to my grandparents' graves. I selected a list for my daughter of what to pay, who to call and what needed to be cancelled. I chose a biodegradable urn for my ashes that was the size and shape of a bowling ball and looked like a planet with a ring around it. Five thousand dollars later, everything was in order.

Whatever I choose to do, I counseled myself, *do not go to pieces and make everyone around me grieve before it is time.* Don't be bitter. Cancer happens. Death happens.

And why *not* me? I had had a long life. I couldn't keep pretending I would live on and on just because I have good genes. I finally felt satisfied I had done as much as I could to save my family from months of work after I died. There was some comfort in knowing I would not be leaving a mess of confusion.

Not everybody is as lucky as my 79 year old grandpa, who had a heart attack and died while sitting in his easy chair watching his favorite baseball team play. A few seconds of pain and it was over. The perfect death, the right age, the Cincinnati Reds game in the background and he had just had a good lunch!

Despite my mom's horrible dying process, she often repeated to me that she was grateful for not having to die alone. I felt grateful, too, for by my side was a wonderful caring daughter, a loving supportive step-daughter, good friends and my sweetheart of twenty years, Nick. I had a roof over my head, Medicare, and my furry kids: George and Momma Blue. I had my community at church, my Pastor and thank God, I had my mind.

Still, every morning I would awaken, pulling myself out of my deep warm dream world and suddenly freeze remembering my new cold reality. *Oh my God, cancer! I have cancer!* It was like putting on a heavy coat that weighed a ton. After I got up, had a shower, drank some tea and fixed my animal kids their breakfasts, I would calm down. I could even forget about cancer for a few minutes while doing some mundane task, then—bam! Like a splash of ice water in my face—*cancer!*

Along with my fear was a heightened awareness of the kindness that surrounded me. Not just friends and family, but the staff at the various doctors' offices I visited were ultra-sensitive to cancer patients. Everyone wanted to help make life easier for us. Even strangers, like clerks in stores, seemed to be extra friendly and sweet to me and they didn't even know I had cancer! Was it my imagination or did I really have a "C" branded on my forehead?

Debra, a friend of mine, said it was Grace and that she had also felt it when she went through her cancer journey of having melanoma. All I knew was that I felt serene most of the time when I wasn't in cold fear. Perhaps it was all the meditating I was doing that made me aware that love was all around. It also helped to talk with people like Debra, who had dealt with cancer twice in her life and was wiser for the experience.

Also helpful were the books Shanen and I were reading written by a modern mystic—Joel Goldsmith (1892-1964). We would read a few pages, stop and discuss what we had read and then close our eyes and try to meditate. I was never a daily meditator, but fear was surely driving me to try harder to become one. After a few months, I felt something shift in my consciousness, as I asked for an awareness of God to come to me.

Meditation was becoming easier for me as I practiced it more regularly. First, I relaxed and let go of tension and thoughts from my monkey mind, then I let go of what was me: ego, personality traits, emotions and all the experiences that made up my identity. If I was lucky, there was a shift in my contemplation, a mental slide into a deeper space of meditation, where I was floating along in a "no mind" state. I went from being the antsy and impatient me, to feeling like I was at peace, lying beside the "still waters that were restoring my soul" (Twenty-third Psalm). I could sit contentedly in the silence forever or at least for twenty minutes. These times of diving deep into my soul through meditation gave me perspective and balance and calmed my panicky heart (see my chapter on meditation).

I also took time to sit outside each evening with all my senses attuned; listening to the world slow down, the birds say goodnight and frogs croak hello. It was healing for me to soak up the peacefulness and beauty of twilight as it turned my garden a lavender blue. Be here now, I told myself. *This is it—this is life!* This moment is all I have, all anyone has, and I am going to pay attention.

CHAPTER 6

Diving Deeper

I love to read inspirational books, especially about people who have had near-death experiences, met angels, seen the Light and returned with good news about life after death. I know some people believe these experiences are just the brain's little trick to peacefully prepare us for death—chemicals released that fool us with sweet illusions. But I believe many of these reported experiences are real and I am comforted by reading them.

Proof of Heaven is such a book by Eben Alexander. It was especially meaningful for me since I heard him speak in person at Charleston's Unitarian Church (sponsored by the local Jung Society). Alexander is a neurosurgeon who was able to decipher what was going on in his body as he experienced deadly bacterial meningitis. His neocortex shut down but his inner adventure continued during his coma. Alexander's near-death experience is the subject of his book, *Proof of Heaven*, which details his supernatural journey while part of his consciousness stayed alert learning about heaven. His story about another realm we exist in after death was and is very reassuring to me.

Another exceptional book that provided me with insights on the possible emotional and mental causes of disease is *The Healing Power of Illness: The Meaning of Symptoms and How to Interpret Them*, by the authors, Thorwald Dethlefsen and Rudiger Dahlke, MD. The subject matter intrigued me as I had long believed there were connections between disease and one's inner life, childhood experiences and personality. I found it fascinating to apply the information to my cancer experience while I was learning how the body, mind and spirit interact.

I learned from this book that often the body will ring the alarm bell first when something is "off" by manifesting a physical symptom. Usually, the afflicted person then runs to the doctor's office to ask the doctor to make the symptoms go away. Sometimes, there is a cure or sometimes the symptom simply moves somewhere else in the body to continue manifesting as another problem. This is commonly referred to as "symptom imperative" or "symptom substitution." You can spend your whole life trying to track down the cause of your problem, running from doctor to doctor, suffering, confused and believing it is strictly physical.

The physical symptom is real *and* may be saying something important to you at another level. That other level may have to be addressed through inquiry, therapy, self-care, prayer, medicine, journaling or dream work. And here is the amazing thing—just maybe that symptom could have a life-changing message for you.

The Healing Power of Illness argues that the body is trying to talk to us. The authors list many illnesses with their connections to what the symptoms are saying. Cancer goes back to love, the authors write, and that seems true to me. Everything goes back to love: unrequited love, betrayed love, lack of love, obsessive love, parental love, unexpressed love; love in all its forms is certainly a major factor in anyone's life.

> I wondered, *if my body was trying to alert me to something unloved in me or my attitude (toward myself), why couldn't it spell it out clearly through dreams, symbols, or intuition? What revelation could be so bad that I had to keep it a secret from myself?*

Therapists will tell you that we keep many secrets from ourselves. I know of people whose symptoms have moved from their neck to their stomach to their shoulder and to their back. Stuck, they go from one doctor to another for various physical problems. The pain goes away for a short time then moves back to their necks, then their shoulders. Like many of us, they run from one doctor to another, spending thousands of dollars, time and energy. This is the plight of many (according to *The Divided Mind* by Dr. John Sarno) and they suffer because they cannot or will not go deeper to explore the psychological cause of the symptom.

Another question I have wondered about is, if once a person figures out the root cause of a symptom and takes action by exploring it, why doesn't this understanding release the symptom? If you had an answer for your suffering, didn't you accomplish the mission of understanding the symptom? From what I've learned, the body develops a pattern of holding on to the symptom, getting into a rut and then the issue becomes stuck in the brain's communication with the nervous system. One has to interrupt the brain's looping process. Some exciting new techniques are coming out that show how working with the brain and nervous system can release these patterns like *Annie Hopper's Dynamic Neural Retraining System.*

Regarding my cancer, I asked myself: *Were there two minds within me—one part wanted healing and the other, my subconsciousness, wanted understanding? Was it using the cancer to communicate with me?* In the book, *Healing Through Illness*, the authors say illness is a path towards healing and growth. "Human illness embodies itself in symptoms. Symptoms are parts of our consciousness's shadow that have translated into physical form."

Shadow work is a Jungian term for bringing forth to consciousness all that we don't want to acknowledge in ourselves. In our shadow lies hidden gold; insights into our character, our development and that which makes up our entirety. The shadow must be incorporated into our personality if we want to become whole. We often despise our shadow's aspects and quite often those are exactly what we despise in others. That's why it is hard to look at them. Dr. Carl Jung said that we humans need to "take the risk of being ourselves." He urged us to take off our masks and learn about the shadow side in order to know ourselves and live an authentic life.

But living an authentic life can be scary. Not everyone

wants to do the work to achieve authenticity. Digging deep into the psyche can stir up lots of pain while it is eliminating self-delusion. We spend years developing strategies that keep us from being honest and keep our mask in place. For myself, one thing I have found out is that I like to be critical of people because by tearing them down in my mind, I feel better about myself. It has nothing to do with their worth, it is about my lack of self-worth. By having learned about this shadow part of myself, I can become more aware of how it does not serve me.

I have been in therapy on and off for years trying to figure out who I am, what made me the way I am and how to eliminate the constant depression I have experienced all my life. Was I willing to go even deeper and examine this cancer diagnosis? Why would some part of me want to develop cancer?

I began by looking at the problems of my knees and legs that I have had since childhood. Were those knobby, sore, cranky knees trying to tell me something as I limped through life? My weak knees kept me from doing certain sports like hiking, tennis, jogging, yoga, and even walking up steps. All I knew for sure was that it all began in my twenties, when I tore some tendons in my left knee while stepping off a curb. That injury never healed properly. Somehow it led to a painful "trick" knee that came and went. I had always resisted surgery in the hopes it would recover. Getting older and gaining weight did not help the situation.

But wait a minute, I reminded myself, *my leg trouble really began when I had a serious sledding accident on a flying saucer disc at thirteen years old.* Someone pushed me at the wrong angle down a steep hill heading the saucer and me towards a tree. I turned my body at the last minute with my left thigh taking the blow. It was a serious break—a fractured femur. Since I was a growing teenage girl and the doctor was concerned that both my legs end up the same length when I reached full growth, he did the conservative thing by using a traction apparatus to keep a slight pull on my injured leg. That would hopefully keep the injured leg growing at the same speed as my good leg.

I was in the hospital for several months, feeling like I was held captive, caged in a metal frame that went around my bed. I was on my back, while my left leg was held in a sling suspended in the air. There was a metal pin inserted through my knee that was wired to weights that pulled on my leg. The whole arrangement was uncomfortable because I was unable to move from that position. Using the bedpan meant pulling myself up to a half-sitting position while holding on to the metal framework overhead. Painful bowel impactions resulted from this awkward position.

One night while I was hospitalized, a male patient across the hall from me, drugged and delirious, broke out of his binding straps that were holding him in bed and rushed into my room naked trying to get onto the window sill to jump out. The sight of a naked man for a thirteen year old was quite startling—plus the fact that I was wired to my bed and couldn't escape. Attendants quickly dragged him out of my room, but I didn't sleep that night listening to him shouting and crying.

I also worried what would happen to me if there was

a fire, since my bed and I were one. A nurse reassured me that someone on duty would take me out of the building on a large elevator that would accommodate the oversized metal contraption I was in. They would take care of me, she consoled, but still I worried every time an alarm went off.

I also learned from my hospital sojourn that love is always around. I was in the adult wing of the hospital (since I was thirteen) with women patients in for hemorrhoid operations. One of my roommates I nicknamed "Minnie-haha" because she laughed all the time. She heard me sobbing one night and came over to my bed and hugged me while I cried on her shoulder. Minnie stopped laughing and gave me some good motherly love. Sometimes we get by on the kindness of strangers—that was another one of my lessons. Yet another was the insensitivity of doctors.

My primary doctor came into my room on morning rounds with a group of male students in tow. There was my young cute doctor, whom I had a crush on, standing with several male interns all gathered around the foot of my bed. He theatrically threw back the blanket to show off his handiwork on my cast. There I lay exposed, a young girl frozen in a white cast which held my legs open wide baring my pubic area upon which I had recently grown a thick bush of hair! I thought I would die of embarrassment as the group of males stood around admiring my "cast."

After three months in the hospital, I was sent home to recuperate on my grandparents' couch for the next few months. The plaster cast was rigid, holding my body firmly in place in a half-seated position. One branch of the hard plaster encasement ran down my injured leg from my rib cage to the tips of my toes and on the right leg it forked from my ribs down below my knee. The heavy white cast wrapped around my stomach and hips with an opening for my eliminations.

The most hurtful part of it all was that I was missing out on the eighth grade, a special year for me since I had been chosen to be a cheerleader. I had also been lucky to get into the class of everyone's favorite teacher, Mr. Lake. I was acutely aware and resentful that I was also missing out on school dances, parties, sportings events and the teenage romances that were beginning to bloom.

There I lay, day after day, watching television, with my grandma as my nurse, cook and bedpan attendant. From the couch, I could see outside our picture window to the street and watch the neighborhood kids walking home from school, laughing and skipping, living another reality from mine. It was a time that I felt I was benched on the sidelines and not in the game of being a teenager.

Two months later, I went back to the doctor where my cast was cut off of my body. It fell away like an empty shell revealing my thin hairy legs which had atrophied and were covered with dead skin. At last, the air could touch them now and I could wash my entire body. I advanced to crutches for the summer and became quite adroit at maneuvering steps. I loved being upright, finally able to sit on a toilet.

When school started in the fall and my girlfriends put on their "cool" shoes—flats, hush puppies, loafers and oxfords, I was off crutches and still limping. I had to wear brown and white corrective shoes that branded me "uncool" for high school. My feet were not yet strong enough to hold me. By winter I was doing better, still limping a little and having pains in my arches since I tossed out those ugly shoes and wore a pair of powder blue flats to school. Each step felt like knives stabbing at my arches, but it was worth it to be "with it."

During this hard time, I pitied myself asking, *why me?* Why was I singled out? Why did I have to give up the best year of my life? Was my sledding collision with the tree really just an accident? Was I accident prone, like my mom told me I was; my accident just a ploy to get her to come home from New York City and leave her exciting life there? I didn't miss her and her dramas that much, so I seriously doubted her theory.

Years later I wondered, *was my mom right?* Did I somehow cause or attract my accident? And how did this help heal anything in the shadows? I knew that my accident made me grow more compassionate because now that I had seen the suffering of others in the hospital, I knew there was another world that my friends in their teen trance were not aware of—a world of pain and suffering.

My lesson from this ordeal was how life could take you from being on top of the mountain (cheerleader) to the bottom of the canyon (crippled) in one second. It was a scary lesson and added to my general fearfulness. Gone was my innocence that my world of teen crushes, rock music and the perfect prom dress were the only reality.

Life pulled the rug out from under me. Decades later,

I started remembering another aspect of the day of the sledding accident and developed a view of what might have been an underlying component. I had started my first menstruation period that day. It was an important day for me since I had been waiting in anticipation of becoming a "woman." I found drops of blood on my panties and proudly put on my first sanitary pad. Maybe that incident held too much energy for me to handle, for it meant I could now become pregnant.

CHAPTER 7

Who to Tell?
What to Tell? When to Tell?

No one knew, besides my immediate family, that I was dealing with the health crisis of cancer. I did not want the word to get out because I dreaded the questions and *everyone* had questions. When I finally began opening up about it, they came flooding in. Where is the cancer? What stage is it? Which hospital system are you in? Who's your doctor? What kind of treatment are you having? Are you going to have chemotherapy? Can I put you on our prayer list?

Mostly, there were questions about what kind of cancer I had and at that time, I did not know. Doctors, after four months, five months, even six months, still didn't know the primary site. That didn't make sense to anyone, or to me. There had to be a primary location because the cancerous lymph node was the evidence.

"You don't have cancer!" One woman accused me when I told her I didn't know what it was called or where it was. I was beginning to feel defensive. Did people think I made this up in order to get attention?

"Are you in pain?" was another question. No, not unless I was being prodded and poked. To close friends, I would tell my "onion under the gas pedal" story, hoping they would understand its impact. I felt conflicted sometimes, as if sharing the incident took away some of the sacredness of it, especially when I got back that look that said, *Poor dear, she's gone bonkers!*

Shanen took the news of my cancer pretty well, I thought, considering she has a tender heart. Later she told me she had her breakdown in private and then armored herself for what she would have to do to help me get through this journey. My step-daughter, Rochelle, and her family came down from Ohio to be with me for a short visit. Nick went into denial, telling his family that I had found a cyst in my groin.

I began to resent the fact that even people I didn't know very well insisted on knowing the details of my cancer. *This is my information,* I thought, *and it's private!* I didn't want to talk about it to just anyone, not knowing how far or changed the information would become— often garbled like the telephone game, "Gossip." Often the questions would come at inappropriate times. *There's a time and a place to talk about such a personal thing,* I felt like screaming, *not from adjacent toilet stalls in the Ladies' Room!*

And no, please don't put me on the prayer list at church. Pray for me if you wish, but I don't want my name on the list made public for every Sunday's church bulletin. As my astute daughter said to me, "All the same names are on the prayer list year after year, doesn't anyone ever get healed?"

I must admit, prayer is a bit confusing to me. I'm still studying the many ways it is practiced. Carolyn Myss, a respected medical intuitive and author, says, "pray as if you are crazy" and "ask for grace." Dr. Larry Dossey says, "prayer is one of the best kept secrets in medical science." Many Christians quote the Bible's references to prayer like, "pray without ceasing..." I have been a part of several prayer groups in my life and received the laying on of hands by a priest. So I am not against it, as long as it is not pleading for something from a Santa Claus-like God.

If prayer is about sending loving thoughts to another, feeling compassion, or praying for their highest good, I am all for it. In *The Infinite Way*, a spiritual wisdom book by Joel Goldsmith, he writes: "...instead of seeking, asking, waiting in prayer, we turn our thoughts inwards and listen for the still small voice." In other words, meditate and enter the stillness within to contact God. Your light will be the best prayer for yourself and others.

My minister, Reverend Ed, was wonderful, respecting the private space I was in. His way of praying for others, he told me, is to support their soul's choices. I liked that. He understood that I considered this a sacred time and I would call on him when and if I needed him. Fortunately, I have a comfortable relationship with him that is based on trust and respect. We both believe that everyone's spiritual journey is to be honored regardless of how it appears to others.

There was one close friend who wouldn't give up interrogating me about my situation. I was annoyed, even though I knew she just wanted to be helpful. Like a dog with a bone, she hung on asking, "just one more question," and after I answered that one, "just one more question." I was getting mad, tiring of explaining my mysterious situation for which I still did not have any definitive answers. Finally, I snapped, "No more!" to her incessant questions. Usually, I wasn't this rude, but I had to draw the line.

Some people wanted to be "helpful" in ways that were not. I did not want to hear about Aunt Tillie, who died a gruesome death of cancer. One friend insisted on explaining to me that if the cancer was in my anal area, I would never be able to sit down again! She was absolutely sure of it because she had a friend who had cancer with surgery in that area who had to stand or lie down for years since she couldn't sit. This "bearer of bad news" also added that this was tough information to share with me, but she was a "truthful" person and felt duty-bound to tell me this awful story. She just *had* to… *YOU DON'T HAVE TO!* I wanted to scream at her as I backed away. Often, I was so stunned at what people thought was appropriate conversation that I was tongue-tied.

Reflecting back, I realize it would have been helpful for me to have had a few quick responses when uncomfortable or inappropriate conversations started regarding my mysterious cancer. "I'm saving that for my book," I could have said humorously, or "I don't want to talk about my health problems right now, but tell me, how you are doing?" Or, "It's a mystery, more will be revealed later and you will be the first to know."

Another question was, what kind of cancer did I have? I felt somewhat protective of talking about it with everyone. I realized that I had the right to decide whom I wanted to tell, when and how much I wanted to tell.

If you are the type who wants to share your story with everyone, that's ok, too—just be true to yourself.

Having cancer did alter some of my relationships. I was stunned at the lack of interest from some of my family and surprised that some close friends were quite attentive while others were not. Relationships are always in a state of flux and cancer is a trigger to many. It's like talking about death; it can be an uncomfortable topic that many people want to avoid. Cancer has affected almost every family and conversations can bring up sad memories. I let go of the expectation that any one of my family or friends would react like I wanted them to—with caring and respect.

I never knew what I would say, since my mood changed from day to day. One day I would be thinking I was going to be fine, then the next day, *Oh my God, I am dying!* How I acted and reacted to others varied according to my mood. Sometimes I might be on the verge of tears, feeling vulnerable or depressed. I advised myself to not feel badly if I was not up for chit-chat and not feel pressured to put up a happy front.

I often have a low tolerance for cheery people, but there were days when I was thankful for those who were so positive about my prognosis. You might want to find a good listener among your friends, someone you can talk to freely about your fears, someone who will not try to minimize your feelings. Your emotions will go up and down: accepting, angry, sad, denying, hopeful, fearful or grieving. Cancer puts you in a fluctuating state of mind that is often determined by your pain level or the latest results of a test.

Speaking to a counselor or therapist is handy during this time to be able to "spill your guts" to, cry as loudly as you want, or pound a pillow in rage. Whatever and whomever you can find to lessen the stress you are enduring is worth the money.

Children in your life will need a special kind of explanation. My daughter prepped my grandson by telling him that his "Mimi" was sick. Then, when he and I were together alone, I asked him if he knew anything about cancer. He is a wise little boy who knew more than I thought. I didn't say too much, but waited to see if he had any questions, so I could follow his lead. I told him he could ask questions of his mom or me at any time. I showed him a pamphlet with a photo of a radiation machine. I explained how it worked which interested his scientific mind the most.

Most children want to know how their lives will be affected. Will they lose their hair, too? Is cancer contagious? Experts advise that children need to be kept in their normal routine as much as possible. Encourage and respect their questions and ask if they have any feelings about what you have told them. In certain circumstances, sadly, you may have to tell them about death, perhaps your death. There are many professionals who can help: a child counselor, a pastor, a family therapist, a minister from the hospital or from your church or a recommendation from a cancer support group member. Keep the children in your life in the loop to the extent that they can handle the information. They may not say much, but those little minds need reassurance.

CHAPTER 8

Green Medicine

Like many people, I became enamored with herbs and their power to heal from back in the day of communes and the book, by Euell Gibbons, *Stalking the Wild Asparagus*. The back-to-nature movement spawned a taste for granola, sassafras tea, brown rice and tofu. We baked our own bread and made our own yogurt. I grew several herbs like comfrey, chamomile, catnip and peppermint for teas. In fact, I still enjoy keeping a few plants around to use for teas and tinctures.

So many medicines come from herbs, trees and flowers (digitalis from the foxglove flower, camphor from the camphor tree, menthol from mint plant) that it's hard to dismiss their power, especially now that we have science to back up their efficacy. More cures from the garden include garlic, thyme, turmeric, pepper, cayenne along with onions, cinnamon, oregano, honey and vinegar. These were the only medicines we had in the cupboard a few hundred years ago.

I experienced the raw power of herbs one night when my mom and I drank big mugs of senna leaf tea to clean out our eliminatory systems. We both had read a book about the build-up of toxins in the intestines and we were sure we needed a good cleaning out. Senna is a well-known herb that causes cramping and is used as an ingredient in many laxatives. Mom was spending an overnight with me and since it was just us, we decided the time was right for our tea party. Luckily, I had some senna in my cupboard.

I was going to make a cup of senna tea for each of us, but instead I made us each a big mug full of it and made it strong, thinking the stronger the better—a big mistake in herbal medicine. Fortunately, we had two bathrooms at the house and that was where we spent the night in cramping hell, moaning condolences to each other through the bathroom registers. Our elimination systems were "cleaned out" all right by this powerful spasmodic! The next morning, we dragged ourselves to the breakfast table looking pale and weak. Mom said that I was so clean and pure she could see my aura!

A better example of the healing power of herbs occurred in Mexico at a natural health resort my daughter and I were visiting. She was nipped in the thigh by a mischievous horse who was trying to grab her purse which had a banana in it. The bite left big teeth marks, red and raised, looking like they would break open and bleed at any minute. The staff raced to the office where a huge jar of arnica root in water set on the counter for such emergencies. Poultices of arnica were applied to her leg and in a few hours, there were some red marks left but most had turned into light bruises. It could have been so much worse.

Herbs can be very dangerous if misused. I once saw a woman on a television show who was headed to an appointment with a plastic surgeon about her nose. She had used an herbal skin cancer remedy on a growth there thinking that if a little would help, then a whole lot must be better. She burned off the tip of her nose with the herbal solution and had to have it reconstructed. Again, the lesson to respect herbs is learned: a little dab'll do ya!

Considering the power of herbs, I was leery when my mom asked me to research herbal poultices to put on her ravaged cancerous breasts. I found information on the internet about pokeweed being a cancer cure and I just happened to have a tall healthy pokeweed bush in my backyard. The recipe said I was to steam the berries with a little water, cool and mash them and place them in a permeable cloth. Putting a poultice of acidic pokeweed berries on mom's open wounds sounded dangerous. I begged off that idea because I really didn't know what I was doing. Good thing too, because pokeweed is highly toxic to the touch and poisonous if ingested. We did venture to apply boiled and cooled cabbage leaves as poultices on her breasts several times, a messy procedure that didn't work. But we didn't stop there.

We tried to cook up some marijuana, hoping it would help Mom with her pain. We weren't able to smoke it because Mom was on oxygen. I didn't cook it correctly, because the plant has to release its special chemical at a certain temperature. I put some butter, a little olive oil and some chopped garlic along with the crumbled weed into a big skillet to simmer. We spread the mixture on crackers and ate it, waiting for a reaction. Hours later, we were still sitting and looking at each other—nothing happened. Stymied, we were afraid to buy any more marijuana since it was illegal in our state.

Mom wasted away from cancer and nothing worked for her pain. She had a reaction to morphine and every other pain killer the doctors gave her. We thought that when things got really bad, there would be drugs, wonderful drugs that would relieve her pain and put her into some tolerable state, comatose maybe, pleasantly floating along in a dream. Sadly, she didn't find relief from any drugs, supplements or herbs.

Many nights I sat with her, as she suffered hour after hour, until I wanted to take her hand, lead us to her bedroom window and jump out. We were only three floors up, so I called hospice instead and their ambulance came to take her to their center while I trailed behind in the car.

My dear mom, so beautiful, so wanting to die and get it over with, was in and out of hospice several times. I did not know you had to be actively dying to have the services of our hospice facility in Dayton, Ohio. Every time she went in for hospice care, she would revive and then be told she must leave. *Die, Mom,* I silently begged her, *end this hell!*

I realized after a few trips that all the attention from the hospice staff enlivened her. One moment she was wailing in agony at home and suddenly there she was, sitting up in bed, regaling the hospice nurses with stories of her glamorous life in New York City. She would be evaluated and asked to leave. I would have to take her home since she was not dying that day. We wouldn't be home long until another night of hell would send us back to hospice and the whole routine would repeat itself.

If only we could have found a painkiller that worked for her. My fear was that floating off on a cloud of morphine might not work for me either. Suffering, even from a paper cut, was not my thing.

About three or four months into my cancer journey, I got a call from a friend, Nancy, who told me that she mentioned my cancer diagnosis to her lawn maintenance man who had been working on her yard that day. He told her about his 91-years old mother, Mary, who was healed from ovarian cancer thirty years ago by using an herbal tonic. He said that his mom was open to sharing her story and he had permission to give out her phone number. Nancy called me immediately to give me this information, saying his mom had taken this herbal remedy when everything else had failed to cure her ovarian cancer. She was still taking a "maintenance" dose and continued to be in good health.

Wow, I couldn't wait to call Mary. No answer. I left my name and number and the reason I was calling. I didn't hear from her for a couple of weeks, so I called again, leaving another message and requesting that she call me back. Again, I heard nothing. Finally, after waiting another few weeks, I decided to make one last call. Mary answered in a cheerful, youthful voice. When I told her the reason for my call, she was happy to tell me her cancer story that happened nearly thirty some years ago when she was in her early sixties.

At that time, Mary said she had tried everything

to cure her ovarian cancer, including two surgeries, chemotherapy, two trips to clinics in Mexico, prayer (she was a Jehovah's Witness) and radium implants. But after all of this, the cancer still had not gone away. Desperate, she called a friend who had a health food store in Atlanta and asked for help. This woman recommended that Mary call another health food store owner in Seattle who might have some recommendations. Mary contacted her and was told about an herbal product called *Vitae Elixxer*. Its creator, Ralph Schauss, a man from Casper, Wyoming, had cured himself of cancer decades ago by formulating this tonic from a variety of ten herbs.

Mary explained to me that she took the tonic drops in water as directed and over a period of eight months it cured her ovarian cancer. "You have to be consistent," Mary said. "That's the key." She reported that she's been healthy ever since and still takes six drops a day as a preventative. "I get a lot of calls from people who want to know what cured me. Even some doctors and scientists call and want to know my story," Mary reported in her chipper voice. "It cured my son of skin cancer, too. He had a melanoma on his arm." She added, "It's helped a lot of friends and family members."

I called to order the tonic, speaking with Ralph Schauss's daughter who had taken over the business after her dad died (not of cancer). Laurie was positive and supportive and had many years of experience with *Vitae Elixxer*. I decided to buy the purple drop formula which was expensive, but lasts for a long time. She assured me she was always available on the phone for counsel and she was good on her word. I received the two bottles of herbal tonic in the mail along with detailed but clear directions. I started with a drop or two in a glass of water, then worked my way up to a few more drops added week by week. I wish I could say I was consistent. I wanted to give it my full cooperation, but after a few weeks, as the dosage increased, I couldn't stomach it. It was *that awful*—just like the canned asparagus had been, and yes, I am a baby about awful-tasting things!

I could not make myself drink the tonic, so I cannot be a witness to its efficacy. Look up the product and decide for yourself. (See vitaeelixxir.com) This is not an endorsement. I was not able to take it for more than three weeks. Maybe if I had put the product in a food like peanut butter or into capsules, I might have been able to get it down. It is expensive and has no scientific studies to support it, but if you talked to Mary, you would be convinced it saved her life.

Another herbal candidate I considered that claims to cure cancer is a tea called *Jason Winters Tea*. Sir Jason Winters healed himself in 1977 from cancer of the jaw using a formula he created which is available for sale on his website. I enjoyed the book, *The Sir Jason Winters Story—From Deadly Cancer to Perfect Health*, a compilation from many sources by Benjamin Roth-Smythe. Winters' original story of healing himself was published in 1980 and is called *Killing Cancer*. All of his stories and travel adventures make for fascinating reading as he covers many healing modalities: herbs, nutrition, attitude, cleansing with coffee enemas, massage therapy, vitamins and much more.

A most remarkable fact about Sir Jason Winters is that

he is considered to be a "walk- in," according to author Ruth Montgomery. This is a New Age term for someone who willingly allows his or her body to be given to another soul to "walk in" and take over. As Montgomery explains in her book, *Threshold to Tomorrow*, the original person just slides on out to another dimension. The name remains the same, but now there is another personality taking over. The mutual agreement for the exchange is for the higher purpose of both souls.

As a young man, while in surgery, Jason reports he decided to leave his body and let another soul primed to do good in this lifetime take over. Ruth Montgomery considers Winters as "...one of the most remarkable human beings I have ever known."

Sir Jason Winters was a remarkable man: a healer, actor, world traveler, tv personality, researcher, spiritual seeker, father and husband. The many herbal products on Winters' website are said to purify the blood so your body can heal itself.

I also experimented with a natural product made from pulverized red raspberry seeds that is full of a compound called Ellagic Acid (EA) which boosts the immune system and stops cancer cell division. Studies done in the late 1990's at Hollings Cancer Center in Charleston, South Carolina show that EA can be effective on a variety of cancers: cervical, breast, pancreas, skin, colon and prostate.

I cannot end this chapter without mentioning the healing properties found in mushrooms. There are over 10,000 varieties of fungi growing all over the world. Chinese medicine has used mushrooms for more than a thousand years in their healing tradition. In the USA, we are just beginning to catch up with studying the healing effects mushrooms have on a variety of ailments, from cancer to boosting the immune system and cognitive function.

Some mushrooms are deadly poisonous, some are hallucinogenic, and some are miraculous and may be the answer to our excess garbage and plastic pollution! Several fungi are being studied for their abilities to secrete enzymes that can dissolve plastic.

I took a mushroom compound during my cancer journey that has had over 30 human clinical trials showing its efficacy in targeting the HPV virus and enhancing immune function. A warning on mushroom use: always be sure they are from a reliable source, and do not list "mycelium powder" in the label. I have discovered that this means they are diluted in potency. Some people find mushrooms too stimulating, others may have allergies. Always do your own research to find reputable companies and invest in quality products.

When the Bible tells us that we are given the herbs and plants for our healing, I believe it. We have only just begun to understand what is out there as Mother Earth's gifts for us. That is why it is so important to keep our jungles, rainforests and natural preserves protected for the benefit of future generations as well.

CHAPTER 9

Psychics
and a Haunting Dream

I was becoming tired of wondering what kind of cancer I had, and since no one in the medical field was coming up with any answers, I decided to do something I normally would never do—contact two psychics to see what they could come up with. I did not call any psychic hot-lines, but reached out to find psychics I felt were reputable.

One was Ann, an established psychic in Dayton, Ohio, who is my daughter's acquaintance from high school days. The other psychic, Gayle, who lived in Asheville, North Carolina, was a friend of a close friend of mine. Each psychic charged one hundred dollars for a two-hour long session which was conducted over the phone—not too expensive and worth a try, I decided.

I was excited when Ann began her reading by giving me the name of my cancer that she received from her "sources." This was exactly the bit of information that I had been wanting and waiting for. Later, when I asked my doctors about the name, I was told it had nothing to do with my cancer's symptoms (and later it was proven as well). Most of the rest of Ann's reading consisted of general information and messages like, "You should teach, you have much to give. Living or dying—it is your choice. You are supported by your guides." Location, location, location was what I was looking for. I was disappointed.

The other psychic gave me information that my cancer was the result of an ancestral connection that led to my father and his boyhood inferiority complex! It was hard for me to see how this created my cancer. I know genetics and ancestral patterns are very hot topics right now, but this was too far of a reach for me. Gayle spent a lot of time talking about her guru who was very important in her life. She insisted I would profit greatly by connecting with this wonderful spiritual teacher. Her enthusiasm bordered on conversion and I wasn't interested.

I tried to use my own kind of psychic intuition; I meditated, listening for that small still voice within to say something. I've gotten a few messages through the years when a voice (not my own) spoke to me in the quiet of my meditation or upon awakening from sleep, but no voice came through when I asked where the cancer was located. I continued to work on it by journaling, studying my dreams and looking at the symbols that appeared in my waking life. I tried a dream process called incubation. Before I went to sleep, I asked my dreams to give me some understanding about the cancer and had the following dream:

I find myself back in the living room of my childhood home where I lived with my grandparents. I see they are in bed in their bedroom. I walk into the living room and find a yellow metal crane—smaller than a real one, but big enough to fill up one half of the living room. I try to move it and accidently knock it against the ceiling. I see that the part of the crane that moves up and down has made a circular yet jagged hole in the ceiling about eight inches in diameter, knocking out the plaster completely. I can see the attic through the hole. Oh goodness, I think, I am responsible for this damage. I'd better take care of it before grandma and grandpa find out. I anxiously look for a stool or ladder to stand on and try to find some spackle to close in the hole. I must do the repair quickly before they see it. I know grandpa will be mad for sure. I entitled this dream: The Cover Up.

I shared this dream with my therapist, describing the yellow crane as a large replica of a toy found in metal erector sets that I remembered boys playing with many years ago. As I was telling my therapist the dream, I was suddenly aware of the name *erector* set, with a part that went up and down, and a chill went through me. He caught the inference too and we exchanged an "aha" expression.

I interpreted my dream like this: The crane's moveable part that goes up and down went too high (out of control) and caused the hole (damage) in the ceiling. I'm to blame. Could this ceiling be the dividing wall between my subconscious and higher consciousness? The attic is also where you store old things you are not willing to let go of or things you might need someday. The most energy-filled dynamic was that it was imperative for me to take care of the damage quickly before anyone found out. I did something wrong and caused the problem. I can view the upper floor through the hole. Could the hole be a wounding or a literal "breakthrough?" I need to get a stool or ladder (something to stand on), spackle and a tool to repair the broken hole. I am anxious to get it done before my grandparents, especially my grandfather, finds out. He will be angry. The hole in the ceiling has opened up a view exposing the dark space above. It was made by something hard that swung up and out of control. I have to hurry. I related this incubated dream to the damage of the cancer to a floor/ceiling of my body. It had something to do with a mistake I had made by being careless with a crane which was part of the erector set. I was to blame. I knew this was a dream of sexual abuse, one of many I have had for the past thirty years.

Could my history of sexual abuse have manifested as cancer? I know that the body has a way of speaking its own language. My dreams and nightmares of childhood sexual abuse were often ignored until I got into dream interpretation. I had dealt somewhat with the abuse in talk therapy and visited a few sexual abuse survivor support groups, but could not identify with the members of the group. In fact, I felt repulsed by their suffering. I noted that many of these women had health problems located in their breasts and genitals. As therapists encouraged me to go deeper, or to keep going to a support group, I refused. My excuse was that I had a more pressing drama with my mother that I needed to deal with. But that's a whole other book!

CHAPTER 10

Eureka!

After several months, my doctors in Charleston still could not find where my cancer was originating from, so I made a second trip to the Mayo Clinic in Jacksonville, Florida—this time with my daughter. There I was again, at the place where you will surely find the latest medical cures, staffed by seasoned doctors and the most efficient system of handling patients you've ever seen. Shanen and I followed their well-timed schedule going from one appointment to the next. We were like the rest of the people walking around the campus with schedules in hand and hope in their eyes, trusting that surely here we would find help. After all, it was the Mayo Clinic!

I arrived at the office of Dr. Dan for the second time. He was sweet, concerned, and as puzzled as all the rest of the doctors I had seen. Once more I felt like a lab specimen, splayed out on a table, exposing my private parts for the exam. You might think I would be getting used to this invasion of privacy by now, but I was not.

For many women, there is an intense psychological

reaction to having a pelvic exam. It is particularly hard for women who have been raped or suffered any kind of sexual abuse. Post Traumatic Stress is there under the covers of the mind and any kind of physical exam of the genital area can trigger it. So much so, that many women don't schedule PAP smears as regularly as they should due to the feelings of shame, fear or pain. The anxiety is so overwhelming that one woman I read about, with a history of rape, asserted that the only way she would permit herself to be examined would be if the doctors put her to "sleep" first. She was having pains in her lower abdomen and needed an exam, but said she would rather die than experience an exam awake!

This is an extreme case, but I don't know of any woman who looks forward to having a vaginal exam. Like a mammogram, it is something that women know they have to do whether they like it or not, but it is not pleasant. I always dreaded my PAP smears and exams from my first one at sixteen. It felt like some medieval torture every time I had to undress and climb into the "saddle" putting my legs up in the air and my feet into the "stirrups."

The metal speculum looked like a torture instrument and felt like one, too. I wondered why they made one size to fit all. No one ever told me I could ask for a smaller speculum, which is available for children and women with small vaginas. In fact, now I am happy to tell women that speculums come in several sizes and to ask for which size they want.

My exams were always complicated by my body rebelling and tensing up as the doctor inserted the speculum and pushed it into my tender inner parts. I tried to disassociate from what was happening by willing myself out of my body to rise up to the ceiling light and hang out there until it was over.

Thank God, the Pap smear has saved many women's lives. I just wish it wasn't so invasive and often painful. The speculum has the same design that has been used for over 200 years. One day we will have something less invasive so that women can do the exam for themselves.

There is a new invention called the "Callascope" that may put the exam into women's hands. This is a small two component unit with a do-it-yourself probe to be inserted by the woman herself. She can see what is going on by watching a small portable screen that shows a picture of her inner parts. If she has been trained, she can spot any problems and refer them to her doctor.

In third world countries, doctors' offices may be a long distance away and this instrument would allow women to do their own exams and get help if indicated. In some foreign cultures, it is forbidden for women to be examined by a male doctor and many women go without a pelvic exam and suffer the consequences. For some of us who are hurt and/or disturbed emotionally by the exam, this device offers a privacy factor and the empowerment of doing the exam yourself. In the future, the Callascope or something similar may become part of every woman's self-care kit.

Women's bodies have always been a mystery because we can't see what is going on down there! All our knowledge comes second hand. A documentary film called, *The (In)Visible Organ,* about the Callascope, is in the process of being made by Andre Kim (2019). There is a twelve-minute version of what will become a 60 minute documentary in the future.

Pelvic exams have always triggered a memory of when I was a little girl about 4 or 5 years old being examined by a doctor I didn't trust. He was the one who gave me my vaccination; that traitor told me he was going to draw a little monkey on my arm and I believed him! And then he took that needle and popped it into my upper arm several times and it hurt! I remember saying to myself: *do not trust him, he lies.*

It was around this time that my mom took me to the same doctor because I had been complaining of soreness in my genital area. There I was, naked and spread out on an exam table under bright lights with my mom nearby explaining to the doctor that I was putting crayons "up there."

"See this?" the doctor asked me, as he pulled up the metal armatures at the end of the table. "Ladies use these when I examine them. I want you to put your feet in them just like the big ladies do."

I was cold. I was naked. There was no escape. I could barely reach the metal foot holders with my toes. The doctor took a quick look, then admonished me, "You mustn't put anything up there." I wondered, *did I put crayons up there?* Yes, I had, but not until after the soreness started.

And here I lay again, a lifetime later, cold, embarrassed and ashamed. I had done something bad, bad, bad and now I must lie here and go through these feelings again. The speculum scraped my tender insides while gloved fingers held me stretched open, lights focused on my private place. It hurt, it-hurt-it-hurt-it-hurt, that little girl in me cried out again. I had to be strong, I was a Big Lady now, not a little girl.

"I see something in the vagina this time," Dr. Dan announced cheerily. "It's a lesion!"

"Take a picture," my quick-thinking daughter directed. He got his phone out and took a photo. We all had a look.

Yes, there it was, a lesion that was the size of a penny and angry looking. Finally, a tumor was making its appearance at "six o'clock," about two inches up into the right side of my vagina. Finally, after all these exams, we had a primary site for the cancer!

"It needs to be excised," Dr. Dan said. "I could do it here at Mayo, but it's surgery and it would be best to have it done where you live. Sometimes the healing afterwards is problematic and you have an excellent hospital in Charleston (Medical University of South Carolina). I recommend you have it done there."

The culprit had been discovered and it was right where I feared it might be: my vagina, a part of my body about which I have such mixed feelings. Shame, anxiety, pride in its responsiveness, worried about its vulnerability, anger, sad that my vagina had been hurt so often and thankful that a baby (my daughter) pushed herself through it to make her entrance into the world. I wondered if other women had such complicated relationships with their genitals.

Thank you, Dr. Dan, mystery solved. I should have felt relieved, but now that the cancer had a location, it became more real. I had seen a photo of it. How long had it been there simmering under the surface of the tissue—since I was that little girl with the sore vagina?

My daughter and I drove back to Charleston with breaking news… a location! Scheduling surgery wasn't hard, even though my surgeon was one of the few women doctors performing oncological surgeries in South Carolina. The line of patients waiting to see Dr. Gray goes around the block. She is very popular because women want a female doctor and her reputation is excellent. A surgery date was set. After months of wondering where the site of the cancer could be, I now knew its location and I wanted it OUT!

CHAPTER 11

Now is the Hour

I was getting nervous—too much time had passed without this cancer being removed. At one doctor's appointment, I asked if the seven months of waiting to discover the location of the cancer was going to affect my outcome. He assured me it was not a problem. Weeks later, I asked the same question again to a different doctor and was told that the more time that goes by, the more chance of the cancer spreading from the lymph nodes to other parts of the body—a process called metastasis. The cancer could metastasize, moving into the liver, lungs, anus, anywhere. What I surmised was true, time was of the essence, but all the delays couldn't be helped. Thankfully, my cancer did not metastasize; that lymph node of mine did its job of containing the cancer cells.

My doctors told me that after surgery the next step would be radiation, followed by chemotherapy. When I heard the word chemo, I shivered and reluctantly decided I'd better go look for a wig. The hospital's gift shop had a private boutique that sold wigs, so I started there.

Nick and I looked over some wigs and talked with the consultant. I have a tiny face and found that most of the wigs would have to be trimmed and re-styled so my face even showed. Wearing wigs is a hot prospect in the subtropical climate of Charleston. I considered the turbans and the scarves that have bangs in front or a fake ponytail sticking out the back of a baseball cap. They looked comfortable and cute, something I could see myself wearing, but I didn't want to make an appointment for a fitting yet. I was still making up my mind about chemotherapy.

My doctors were all saying that the combination of radiation and chemo was the best weapon they had to make sure my cancer was eradicated. Chemotherapy, they informed me, would increase my chance of survival according to the statistics.

I researched chemotherapy, which I already knew poisons the body while it is killing the cancer cells. It sounded ghastly. Even though the statistics tell you how many people survive after chemo, they don't tell you what condition these people are in for the rest of their lives.

My doctors conferred and asked me again if I understood that the one-two punch of radiation with chemotherapy would give me the best chance for recovery. I wondered, *am I crazy not to have chemo?* I decided to get a second opinion, even though it felt like a betrayal to my medical team.

Being new at all this, I didn't realize that a second opinion is always in order every time there is a major health decision involved. Medical protocol informs us to tell our doctors we are getting a second opinion; it's a common practice and they are accustomed to it. Seek out a doctor who is not in your doctor's practice or department. Check to see if your insurance covers a second opinion. It should. Also, talk to the staff at the second doctor's office and find out what information they want you to bring to the appointment. They will need to see your original doctor's diagnosis and copies of the tests and scans you have had so far. These can be hand-carried or faxed to them.

Be prepared to hear something that might confuse, complicate or even contradict your original path—that's the hardest part of getting a second opinion. Educate yourself, be responsible for getting information for the decision you are making; it is your life and you don't want to look back and say if only—if only I had asked more questions or gotten a second opinion. (See Chapter Twenty-five, *A Whole Brain Approach to Decision Making.*)

For my second opinion, I decided to talk to the radiation doctor at another hospital hoping she might say, "Oh, let's just cut out that tumor and you'll be fine." Instead, after looking at all my records and test results, she said, "I agree with your doctors, after surgery, you need radiation and chemotherapy." I felt trapped.

I conferred again with my surgeon, Dr. Gray, who introduced me to Dr. Cope, the radiologist who was to be the other part of my team. Dr. Cope did not look very seasoned, with his wrinkle-free face and signature silk bow tie, but he turned out to be an experienced radiologist who gave me the respect and kind attention

I needed with this very personal cancer. I watched him carefully, noting how he examined me and talked to me.

I wasn't sure how one evaluates a radiologist's skills at designing the correct angles of the radiation beams. I once asked him if he had gotten good grades in geometry and he said with a smile, "No, but I was good at physics. That actually is better." He had my life in his hands and I hoped he was a genius.

It turned out that Dr. Cope and I developed a good relationship. He was a sensitive man who understood he was treating my private parts and that I might have some feelings about that! He warmed up to my off-beat sense of humor and enjoyed some of the ploys I used to keep my mind off of being examined. During one exam, I asked Jen, his nurse, who was always there holding my tense hand, to join me in a rousing version of "She'll Be Coming Round the Mountain When She Comes." The duet worked to keep me distracted from the painful exam. She and I had a good laugh and I saw a flicker of a smile come over Dr. Cope's face.

On my next visit with my surgeon, Dr. Gray informed me about the procedure she would soon be performing on my vagina. "During the process of the surgery, there is a chance that your sphincter could be damaged and you would then require a colostomy bag, but it's not likely to happen," she explained. But what if it did? I would have to live a very compromised life! *Well*, I reconciled myself, *many people deal with colostomy bags and are able to go on with their lives*. I decided I could, too.

An appointment for surgery was made and I was told the operation would only take a few hours as an out-patient. As she went over this with me, I noticed Dr. Gray wore a gold cross around her neck. She asked me if I would like the name of a Christian-oriented therapist she knew who was very good. "Sure," I said, "give me her card." I liked having available all the resources I could, Christian, Buddhist or otherwise.

As we came to the close of our conversation about surgery, I decided to take a chance and tell Dr. Gray a little bit of my story of childhood abuse. I'm sure she has heard all this before, from many of the women patients she's treated over the years. I felt relieved to have told her something personal about myself. I wanted to be seen as a human being and I wanted to explain why I overreact during the exams. At last, I was moving toward my surgery date and hoping I hadn't lost too much time.

CHAPTER 12

The Other Shoe Drops

June 17th was the day of the surgery to remove the tumor from my vagina. It would take only a few hours as an out-patient, scheduled very early on a Monday morning. I was to be at the hospital ready to be prepped at 5:45 a.m. My sweetheart wanted to drive me, relieved that he could do something substantial to help me. Nick was my rock, affirming that I would be fine and live many more years with him. He had helped me through two knee replacements in the past few years and I had been there for him for five heart bypasses. Thank God, we had each other.

It was totally dark with no morning light at 4:30 a.m. and chilly, even though it was the middle of June. I felt groggy and grumpy. Nick had not driven at this hour in years and we were shocked at the low visibility—not even moonlight. We drove out of my neighborhood in a somber mood, headed to downtown Charleston. At a fork in the road before the bridge into Charleston proper, he blanked out; suddenly panicking and not able to make up his mind which way to go.

Instead of taking the correct road to the left, Nick wavered and drove right up into the middle of a little island where the road sign is located. Jolted, we sat there for a few moments, shocked. Then, he started to back up the car to get into a position to take the road to the left. I looked into my side mirror and panicked, seeing the bright lights of oncoming morning traffic quickly approaching from behind us.

That's when I lost my temper and started shouting at him, "Stop, don't back up!" We were sitting ducks. "Keep going to the right," I ordered. "We can get downtown from the other lane." I wondered how he could have gotten so mixed up on a street he took several times a week to his part-time job.

The hospital is located in an old neighborhood with many one-way streets and vintage street lights. Once more, Nick became confused and drove down a one-way street going the wrong way! Again, I found myself raising my voice, yelling, "Stop!" And again, we almost had an accident with a car coming directly at us—we were in the wrong lane! There was a wet sheen on the pavement and neither one of us could see the markings on the dark streets. It was beginning to feel like a nightmare.

Finally, we arrived at the hospital's entrance, just in time for my check-in. "I'll wait in the reception area for you," I told him. "After you park the car, just come on in." What I really wanted to scream was, "You endangered our lives three times. We could have been killed in an accident!" Nick acknowledged my directions and apologized for his driving. Thank God, I nodded acceptance of his apology and didn't say anything sarcastic or mean. So far, our morning had been bad enough.

I walked into the hospital's large reception room and checked in at a kiosk. Much to my surprise, I was called to the desk immediately then told to go to the second floor for the next step. "Please tell my companion where I went," I asked the receptionist. Things were moving faster than I had expected.

Upstairs at another check-in, I asked another nurse to tell Nick, when he arrived, where they had taken me. I had no idea what was taking him so long. My surgery was happening in a few minutes and I wanted to see him before I went "under the knife."

I was taken to a cubicle where all the last prep was done by a commanding head nurse who wore a military badge indicating she was a sergeant. "Something's wrong," I kept telling her, insisting, "Please keep trying his cell phone."

Convinced I was just worried about my surgery, Nurse Sergeant, accustomed to taking control of hysterical patients like me, said, "He's okay, dear." I felt a foreboding and asked, "How do you know?"

"I know *in my heart* he's okay," she soothed, as if she were psychic. Oh, how wrong she was.

"Let me call my daughter," I asked at the last minute before they wheeled me away. "Something's wrong," I said to Shanen, waking her up. It was still very early. "I can't reach Nick and I don't know what's going on. I think you'd better come to the hospital."

I was wheeled into surgery, shifted onto the operating table and... that's all folks! I like being knocked out. I have been told that a lot of other people like it, too. For a time, there are no worries, you are gone. And then there you are back inside yourself, knowing something terrible has happened to your body and YOU WEREN'T EVEN THERE!

I was coming out of anesthesia. *What had happened? Where was Nick?* My daughter told me she had been calling him repeatedly. Finally, a nurse answered his phone and said, "Nicholas is here with us in ICU. He's had a heart attack! Come right now!"

Bystanders reported that Nick drove to the hospital's parking garage, parked the car, got out and fell to his knees. He collapsed instantly of a heart attack and brain embolism. Emergency help was right there at the hospital and he was rushed to the ICU, but it was too late.

I was jarred out of my post-surgical dream state and my daughter and I were off racing from one building to another in the huge hospital complex. We ended up at the Intensive Care Unit being led to a room where Nick was lying on a table, his clothes ripped partially off his body, plugged into a mess of wires that were keeping his heart pumping. I knew immediately he was gone. Gone. We stood there in shock, looking at him for a long time. Finally, I leaned in close to him and whispered my goodbyes in his ear.

Our crazy ride to the hospital that morning was now very clear. Nick's miscalculations of what street to turn on, almost three accidents, the recent months of his not feeling well, the appointment a week ago at his doctor's where I begged the doctor to do something to help him with his weak legs and non-existent energy, Nick was dying even then. My sweetheart of twenty years was dead.

I couldn't fathom it. I still can't. I go over that morning, trying to put the pieces together. We could have been killed driving downtown or we could have run into someone and killed them. I consider a quick death a blessing and so did Nick. Many times, he told me that he was looking forward to the next chapter of life after death, curious and excited, to see what happens. That was a comfort to me.

After a few days of recovering from my surgery, I went to his apartment and gathered some of the personal things that I had given him over the years: Christmas ornaments, books on cooking and world history, the dog bed he kept in case my dog, George, needed a place to nap, the photo collage of us on the beach and the souvenirs from Mexico were all stacked in a corner to be picked up later when I felt better.

His family arrived from out-of-town and handled everything, thank goodness. A few days after his death, one of his daughters brought me a surprisingly heavy wooden box with half of his ashes in it, keeping the other half for their family memorial. I placed the box under my bed and took it out a few times in the following weeks, looking at it, trying to get my mind around the fact that in this heavy box was what was left of Nick.

Two months later, I organized a sweet, simple ceremony of releasing his ashes into the river. A small group of close friends gathered at one couple's home located on the river and we enjoyed lunch together while sharing stories and memories of Nick. Then we all followed a path behind their home to a pier on the water. A gentle rain began to fall, which chased away the fishermen, so we had the dock to ourselves. After a final toast, I opened the box, took out the plastic bag and gently shook out the ashes, letting them drift down to the current below. It was Nick's last trip to his beloved ocean. Bon Voyage, dear man.

Postscript

I had this dream about a month before Nick's death:

> *Nick, Shanen and I are sitting on the top of a very high cliff at the beach. The cliff is located hundreds of yards back from the waves. Suddenly, Nick gets up, walks behind us, turns around and takes off running at top speed towards us. When he gets to the edge of the cliff where we are still sitting, he takes off into the air in a swan dive. Much to our shock he dives to his death.*

I told Shanen my dream (I did not tell Nick) and said, "Nick may die soon. It will be sudden and shocking."

CHAPTER 13

"Heck No" to Chemo

I had counted on Nick to help me through the next step in my healing journey; a summer of trips downtown to the cancer center for radiation treatments. He had been so eager to support me. Now that he was gone, I would not only miss him, but I would need to replace him and find others besides my daughter to fill in if I needed help with the driving. Even though the doctors made it sound like a nice little get-together, I knew radiation treatments would be no picnic.

"You'll get to know our staff and they'll be friends you'll see every day," the nurse reassured me, as she set up my radiation schedule. "Some people work right on through radiation and chemo," she cheerily added. *Not if they have a choice*, I thought.

I knew that radiation is a killing machine and has many nasty side effects. I was putting my life in the radiation team's hands. I prayed they were experienced enough to aim those radiation beams right where they were needed, by-passing all the important organs and parts I really wanted to keep.

The night before my first radiation appointment, I tried to relax and clear my mind. As I often do when seeking guidance, I looked at my personal library shelves and ran my hand over the books waiting for one to speak to me. I had a set of books my mom bought in the 1960's called, *The Life and Teaching of the Masters of the Far East.* I had ended up with them after she died, but never read them. There were five volumes and I picked out Volume 3 to look for a confirmation that what I was about to do the next day was the right choice.

I lay on the couch, readying my mind for what comfort was to be found in this small book by Baird Spalding. I opened it randomly to a page and began to read: "...any resistance to this energy immediately magnifies it...do not set up any resistance to this light. It will pour out its healing balm... this *radiation* of cosmic light vibrations generated in the great Cosmos, this *radiation* is the great universal light energy that sustains all..." Well, all right! In the space of the next four pages, the word "radiation" was mentioned *eleven times*! Not radiate or radiating, but the word *radiation*. I had my assurance, thank you.

The next day I drove myself to the hospital for my first radiation treatment. I never drink more than a glass of water per day, but was now instructed to glug down 24 ounces of water 30 minutes before I left the house to go to my appointment. I had to hold that water in my bladder while I drove twenty minutes downtown, parked, walked to the building, then waited sometimes up to fifteen to twenty minutes to be called in. Then, continue to "hold it" as I lay on a table and the radiation machines whirred above my head for another fifteen minutes. Then and only then, could I run to the toilet without leaking urine somewhere along the way. Oh boy, what a challenge!

This water torture had to be done before every treatment because a consistently full bladder was of utmost importance. Filling it with the same amount of water every time would keep my bladder in the same place for every treatment, out of the way of the radiation beams.

There were other techniques the staff used to keep me in the best position for the deadly rays to miss what didn't need to be burned up. Two tiny dots were tattooed on my midriff which were used to line me up for the beams. The other positioning trick was a fiberglass mold they made of an impression of my buttocks, which I slipped into every time I lay down on the table. This mold was a perfect fit for holding my body still and in the right place (kind of reminiscent of my plaster body cast I had when I broke my leg). I climbed on the table and wiggled myself into it for every treatment. Then two nurses would fine tune my position even more by pulling and tugging at the sheets I was lying on to gently jostle me a half inch this way or that, to get me just where I needed to be. That sheet tugging technique didn't seem very high-tech, but they reassured me they had it down to a science. All this "fussing" to line me up was frustrating while I was inwardly crying out, *Hurry, I have to pee!*

Once they had adjusted me to their satisfaction, they left and observed me from a window on the far side of the treatment room where they were safe from those deadly radiation beams. For the next fifteen minutes, I entered a self-induced trance while big machines whirred in a circle over me. I would relax and drift off, thinking about what I had read the night before—that little book affirming the healing power of "radiation." *Cosmic or not, I mused, radiation could save my life.*

CHAPTER 14

The Waiting Room

Sitting in the waiting room before my radiation treatments was the toughest part of radiation therapy for me. There sat the old and young, waiting their turns on the roulette wheel of life and death. A young girl about thirteen with one eye bandaged sat glumly in a wheelchair with her mother by her side. I thought of my own daughter at that difficult age and how the worst thing we had to confront was her not being chosen for the cheerleading squad. Thank God, we never had to support her through a serious illness. I saw how the teen's mother was acting—casual and "cool" while I knew her heart was breaking. She was keeping it all together for the sake of her daughter.

Another young woman, who was taking her turn to go to the treatment room, insisted on getting out of her wheelchair and trying to walk down the long hall without any help. Her mother walked behind with the wheelchair, watching her daughter struggle, so weak but determined to do it. Finally, one day I saw she could only make it half-way before she fell back into the wheelchair.

Unable to meet the challenge she set for herself, she dropped her head in disappointment and let her mother push her the rest of the way. My heart broke for these young people and their parents.

One afternoon an older man in the waiting room began to cough and then bleed from his throat incision. Putting his handkerchief to his throat, he apologized to us sitting around the room, as if he had offended us. *Oh no*, we assured him, helpless, hurting for him, not sure of what to do. Thankfully, a nurse was alerted and ran out to take care of him.

Another glimpse of the waiting room was a really odd vision of three older men sitting in a row, waiting for radiation with parts of their cheeks replaced with what looked like plump flesh taken from their buttocks. Surgery made their "cheeks" smooth—no more wrinkles—a small consolation.

I kept my eyes down as much as I could, concentrating on *People* magazine or reading a book I brought with me. Sometimes I looked up and was sorry I did. There was one patient wheeled in who was scarred all over what was left of her body. She was minus an arm from the elbow down and one lower leg. Her face was scarred, too, and she had no eyelashes or eyebrows and was wearing a colorful turban over her bald head. To my surprise she had applied bright blue eyeshadow. That touch of makeup to brighten up her scarred face broke my heart. She, too, was getting radiation treatments and going in all "prettied up." She inspired me not to show up looking like something the cat dragged in.

The first seven or eight treatments were easy on me

and I grew to respect the three nurses who helped me. They were always light-hearted and caring. The whole process was a hurried deal, not much time for chit-chat since they were on a tight schedule working with one patient after another, like an assembly line. Our brief conversations allowed us to establish a small connection. One nurse shared with me that she was getting ready for her wedding day and showed me a photo of her soon-to-be husband. She was so beautiful and he, so handsome, that I wished I could be on the guest list on their big day just to see her in her dress. Ironically, I unexpectedly met the groom's mother a year later and got to see the wedding photos of this stunning couple. Small wish granted.

I was warned by Dr. Cope that radiation would cause skin burns eventually and some nausea and diarrhea… but he reassured me that not everybody has those symptoms. I was reminded once again that many people work right through their treatments. I was so thankful I didn't have kids to care for or a job I had to keep up with. I could go home and nap after treatments.

After a few months, I began to suffer the symptoms of radiation: burned skin in and around my genitals, my butt crack was splitting open with tiny razor-like nicks in the skin, nausea, cramping and explosive diarrhea hit me without warning. I was beginning to see what radiation could do.

The trips downtown to the cancer center got harder as I grew weaker and my body just didn't want to go. My trips were easier if I had someone to drive me when my daughter wasn't available. Just having someone to talk to during the ride was a relief. I asked my friends to please wait for me in the lobby instead of the waiting room. I didn't want them to become as traumatized as I was by the sight of the sick patients there.

My summer consisted of daily trips downtown to the cancer center for six weeks (thirty treatments in all) with Saturdays and Sundays off for good behavior. The diarrhea was constant in the beginning and once I even lost my bowels in Home Depot's parking lot.

I was helpless that afternoon when I felt what was starting to happen. I knew I could not make it to the back of the store to the restroom, so I ran to my car with feces leaking down my legs and out the bottom of my pants. I jumped into my car and took off for home. It's humbling to sit in your own shit while poking along in five o'clock bumper to bumper traffic—and painful, too. I wanted to scream, *Let me through you idiots! I'm sitting on molten lava!*

The worst pain was urinating what felt like razor blades and pooping glass shards. One night that pain had me literally running through the house screaming. I was out of my mind. I had never before tried to physically outrun pain. It didn't work—there was no escape. Thankfully, it was never that bad again.

I managed my bowel movements as best I could, following my doctor's helpful suggestions. A medication controlled the diarrhea so I was able to go out and about with some security. I might then suffer constipation, but at least the Home Depot explosion didn't happen again. There were pads or disposable diapers I could wear for added protection. I was constantly managing my eliminations, trying to find a balance between too much or too little control.

I found that I could no longer eat spicy food or the amounts of fruit and nuts I once enjoyed. Too much roughage. The nurses gave me an aloe gel to put on my body for the radiation burns and I ordered a calendula gel which I used along with a lavender hydrosol spray to soothe and heal. I took long soaks in the bath with baking soda (never Epsom salt, bubble baths or fragrances that are irritating to burned skin) and I discovered that using a hair dryer to dry the skin around my delicate area was much better than the chafing of drying with a towel.

Countdown: day after day for six weeks and finally, radiation was over. With the last treatment, there was a bell to ring in the waiting room to announce the completion of radiation treatment. Everyone in the waiting room applauds in congratulations and a certificate is given, signed by the three nurses who have been your attending team. I didn't want to ring the bell; it felt like I would be tempting fate. Besides, it didn't feel right ringing the bell while looking out on those people in the waiting room who were wondering if they would make it through their next treatment. Finally, my daughter suggested to me that it was not a victory over cancer, but a celebration of the fact that I had finished the 30 treatments. I half-heartedly rang the bell.

CHAPTER 15

Survivors and Supporters

Only one percent of female cancers are related to the vagina, making it a rare form of cancer. I asked my doctors if there was a support group for women with vaginal cancer, like there was for breast and ovarian cancer patients. Unfortunately, there was nothing I could find at the hospital or elsewhere. I called some helplines for cancer support and located a nonprofit group called *Friends for Life* located in Louisville, Kentucky. Their organization connects one with someone who has survived a similar cancer.

When I called their office, they were only able to give me the names of two women in their files who had experienced vaginal cancer. One survivor was Pam, who dealt with vaginal cancer twenty years ago and the other was Sue, who had dealt with cancer thirty years ago. *Long term survivors,* I thought, which was encouraging, but their treatments were done so long ago I wondered if they would be relevant for me in 2019.

I initiated phone calls to both women. The first woman I reached was Pam, who told me that chemotherapy was so horrible she wouldn't wish it on her worst enemy. She explained that she had many after-effects from it like neuropathy, leukemia and scar tissue. She now walks with a cane. All this, she believed, resulted from chemotherapy.

The other woman, Sue, stayed in contact with me for the whole year. As I learned her story, I told Sue she should write a book on her experience of vaginal cancer.

Sue's story began over thirty years ago with the birth of a baby boy with brain cancer. She was with her child every minute of his long stay in the hospital as he underwent painful treatments. One night, she called out to God, begging that she be the one with cancer instead of her baby. "Be careful what you pray for," she told me, for her prayers were soon answered. Her son was healed and she got vaginal cancer.

Thirty years ago, treatment for vaginal cancer was brutal. Sue said that radium "seeds" or inserts were placed in her vagina through metal pipes or rods. The pain was so bad she carried a washcloth to the hospital to bite on.

Through the years, she had colon cancer twice and the resulting scar tissue from that and from vaginal cancer has filled up her lower torso. "I am amazed I have lived this long," Sue told me. At sixty-five, she is often in discomfort and incontinent, but says she has lived a full life with grandkids to care for and an enjoyable job. She believes cancer will eventually return, if it hasn't already, to claim her life. But she refuses to go to the doctor to find out her condition.

Sue stayed in contact with me and cheered me

on. I had no one else to talk to who had experienced this kind of cancer. I kept reminding myself that her treatments were done decades ago and they couldn't be that barbaric today. The fact that she survived for so long was encouraging to me.

I asked Dr. Cope about those inserts and he said that containers of radium are still used in some cancers in order to best target the cancerous areas. I was so thankful I didn't have to have this type of treatment.

There are two types of intracavity inserts: LDR brachytherapy, which places radioactive material inside a cylinder that is inserted into the vagina; a procedure experienced in a hospital setting which may require an overnight or two. The other is HDR brachytherapy, the same process, but done as an out-patient at the hospital and inserted for a shorter period of time.

I read about this type of therapy in *Bone: Dying into Life*, a book by Marion Woodman. It is a journal of her experience with cancer of the uterus, which involved both regular radiation and intracavitary brachytherapy. When uterine cancer struck in 1993, she was around 65 years of age. Woodman used dreams, imagery, body work, alternative health modalities, self-inquiry and traditional medicine to fight for her life. She described being packed with radium inserts as the worst pain she had ever felt in her life; something she endured only with the help of Demerol for the agonizing two days she spent in the hospital.

A treasury of feminine wisdom, Woodman, with her gifts of being a Jungian analyst, author and workshop presenter, approached healing her cancer with everything she had: courage, intelligence and a lifetime of working with the hidden mysteries of the mind, spirit and body. I admired her for standing up to the harshness and dismissiveness of doctors toward her as an older woman. I related to her because she worked with symbols and dreams, going "deep" to find out more about this conflict within her body and how she could heal it.

Just as soon as she had the uterine tumor defeated through radiation, another tumor was found in her sacral area in a location that the doctors said was inoperable. Again, she had to go deep into the "bone" of her existence to figure out what was needed by her body to heal.

She realized that at this time in her life she was a Crone, an archetype for the old wise woman. The task of the Crone is to balance continued passion for life while surrendering to death. She admitted that with age she felt detached and had lost her creative edge which she believed kept her tied to life. "With that loss of creativity, went my power to heal myself," she wrote.

In her book, *Bone: Dying into Life*, Woodman described her medical treatment along with some of the natural therapies she used. With her second cancer diagnosis came her doctor's prediction of two months to two years to live. She wrote her doctor a letter saying she was moving on and wanted a new doctor who would see her without the word "dead" branded across her forehead. She wished him well and acquired another doctor. After more tests and more waiting came the good news that her back tumor was benign. Marion lived another 25 years, dying a few months before she turned ninety in 2018.

I was fortunate to have found this remarkable book

that gave me a vision of how an enlightened soul dealt with cancer and impending death. Marion explored her shadow side and pursued both medical and alternative medicine paths. She also used her dreams, creativity and intuition. At the end of her book, in a symbolic act, she chose to continue the dance of life. She described the turning point happened at a party she went to with her husband where there was great live music and dancing going on. She was weak and didn't know if she could do it or not, but cancer wasn't going to stop her. She felt the music and got out there on the dance floor and danced!

Part Two

CHAPTER 16

What's Going on Down There?

M any women are not sure about what goes on "down there." It was only in the 1960's that women were encouraged to get a mirror and take a look! Some women don't know their own anatomy even after having a baby. We have been taught that this private place is to be kept in the shadows, as if it were shameful.

I remember once talking to a coworker about our bodies and she told me, "I tell my little girl not to let anyone touch her pocketbook!" I replied, "Pocketbook, what's that?" "Vagina!" my friend answered as if I had been raised in the dark ages. Then, I remembered my grandmother using equally confounding words such as "hocus pocus" for my genitals. Maybe my friend's little girl grew up thinking she could use her vagina to carry her money and keys. No wonder we may grow up confused!

Here is some basic information I wish I had known growing up, along with good sex information. The vagina is the opening to a woman's most sacred place where babies are created and grow for nine months. The sperm is ejaculated into this muscular tube that connects the uterus to the outer genitals. It is the entryway to the uterus and ovaries where life begins. The outer lips (labia), the secretions (from the Bartholin gland), the tissues, the underlying muscles, nerves, the length and width of the canal, and the shape and scent are unique to each woman. It is a quite nicely designed system.

The vulva is where the clitoris is nestled between the outer lips and that clitoris has more nerve cells than a penis! The genital area is kept moist by lubricating glands. Because it is warm, it creates the perfect environment for bacterial or yeast overgrowth. Some lucky women go through life without problems in their genitals, while others suffer from burning, itching, atrophy, infections or sexually transmitted diseases.

HPV is one STD that has proven to have direct connections to cancer. Human Papillomavirus, also known as genital warts, is spreading like wildfire. Recent commercials on television dramatize young people asking questions of their parents: "Did you know? Mom? Dad? If you knew there was a connection to cancer, then why didn't you give me the HPV vaccine?" It seems tragic for a young person to be faced with this virus that doesn't have a cure, and then to find out that it can be spread to others adding to the already high risk of sex. This connection of HPV to cancer of the genitals for both sexes also has a higher incidence of cancer in the mouth and throat for males.

There are over 150 strains of HPV related viruses, each classified as high or low risk. It is now the most common sexually transmitted disease. Some cases of HPV come with genital warts that are visible. At least 50% of sexually active people will get HPV and many, like me, will not even know they have it. I was shocked to learn that I had HPV and could have had it for decades.

HPV can be diagnosed by a specific test taken during a gynecological exam. Unfortunately, there is no cure for HPV and there are three million new cases every year.

The new vaccine for HPVcan help prevent cervical, anal and throat cancers. The vaccine can be given from age nine to twenty-six, but the preferred age is around eleven or twelve years old. It consists of three shots done over a six months' time period.

Wearing a condom doesn't always offer protection. HPV is *not* spread through contact with bodily fluids like semen but through skin-to-skin contact.

Also known as genital warts, this virus can show up visually for women as small growths on the labia. A gynecologist can treat these in an office procedure and sometimes they don't come back again. Some lucky people are actually able to clear the virus. It is not known why.

Many years ago, when I asked a doctor if I, as an older woman, should continue to have vaginal exams and Pap smears, I was told, "If you have never had any serious concerns in that area then no, not necessary." I liked that information because I hated those exams. However, later, another doctor told me that every woman should have a pelvic exam every year no matter her age and we must be just as vigilant of our breasts.

Shockingly, every year 300,000 women get some

form of breast cancer and 40,000 die. That doesn't tell the rest of the story of those "cured" women who live with the side effects of chemotherapy and radiation: painful scar tissue, damage from radiation burns, fatigue, lymphedema, chemo-poisoning, weakened immune systems, neuropathy and emotional duress for the rest of their lives.

How can we protect ourselves from cancer? There must be something we can do to prevent it. Watch what we eat? Stay out of the sun, never eat sugar, smoke, drink, have sex or have an x-ray? We are always spraying some chemical on or around us and we are always breathing in pollution. All of our food and its packaging are loaded with chemicals. Some of the conflicting information can be maddening as one expert extols the value of sunshine and another warns never be in the sun without sunscreen and then the third expert believes that the problem is the sun-screen causing the cancer!

Mammograms are now digitized and technically better than in the past, but how many do we need starting at forty and going to seventy years of age or more? That's a lot of radiation. There are many women who believe that mammograms are overrated. I tried thermography once instead of a mammogram to avoid the extra radiation. The heat scan showed a hot spot on my right breast. I was told to come back in six months and they would look at it again. Six months! That wait didn't feel right to me, so I ended up going in for a mammogram after all.

A small benign lump was removed from my breast at my doctor's office. If something does show up in the thermograph, you still have to follow up with your medical doctor and you may end up having a mammogram anyway. Research thermography and decide for yourself.

We must take responsibility for our health. Hands-on exams easily performed in the shower can familiarize us with our bodies. We can check on a regular basis for any changes in our breasts or vaginas. Two of my friends found their breast cancer tumors doing self-exams. Their self-care saved their lives.

Check yourself out for any lumps, bumps or mole changes. Look everywhere, even between your toes! Be sure your doctor also examines anything suspicious and refers you to a dermatologist once a year for a routine full body skin exam. Currently, dentists do oral cancer exams as part of their routine, examining your tongue, throat, roof of your mouth, inside of the cheeks and they should feel around your neck and jaw for anything suspicious. If they forget, be sure to remind them.

A good breast exam is hard to find. The only good one I ever had was by a woman doctor who took her time and wasn't afraid my breasts were going to bite her. Make sure you are examined sitting up and lying down. The physician's fingers should go around each breast in concentric penny-sized circles, checking the armpits and going up to the collar bones. The nipples and areolas should be examined for any changes. Interesting fact: very rarely do men get breast cancer, but if they do, it is more deadly.

Soap up your breasts in the shower and get going, ladies! Hang your how-to instructions (available from your doctor) on your shower head and follow the steps.

Get to know your breasts and assure them, "Girls, you are in safe hands!" That goes for our vaginas, too.

As females we go though many more changes with our bodies than do men. We have our periods and hormonal fluctuations, cramping, flooding, back pain and worry. We go through perimenopause and menopause, with its fatigue, hot flashes, vertigo, mood swings and sweats. After having a baby, once more we have pain, tears that may injure or weaken the vaginal tissues, tenderness and hemorrhoids. Our vaginas have been painfully stretched in childbirth from the size of an almond to a football. If men had to push an eight-pound watermelon out of their rectums, then birth control would be a no-brainer!

CHAPTER 17

Searching for Answers

After all these decades, we still don't know what causes certain cancers, although lots of theories have been offered. In her book, *Cure for All Cancers*, Dr. Hulda Clark claims cancer is caused by parasites. That's right, parasites! Who knows, maybe she will be proven right. I am reminded of my dream of parasites falling off my body a few months before my cancerous lymph node appeared. I have read that our bodies are full of bacteria, microbes, micro-flora and parasites that exist in balance for most of our lives.

Dr. Matthias Rath believes collagen is the key to fighting cancer and the body must be supported by proline and lysine to keep the immune system fit for the fight. He writes most convincingly about the value of collagen and his booklet *Cancer*, from his cellular health series, which has many illustrations of cells and how collagen protects them.

Some researchers say that cancer is a repair mechanism instigated by cells that are triggered by an injury. Lack of nutritional support for your immune system is another theory or too many toxins in the body is another conclusion. There is one theory that says we all have cancer cells in our bodies just roaming around, waiting for the immune system to weaken so they can seize the opportunity to pounce. Like a gang of wild teenagers looking for trouble, they circulate, looking for a weak spot in the body to attack.

We do know that smoking causes lung cancer, tobacco chewing causes cancer of the mouth, and now we know that HPV can cause cancer of the throat, genitals and cervix. For my mother, estrogen taken over decades preceded her breast cancer. She trusted a doctor who told her that taking estrogen along with progesterone was a safe natural way to keep everything in balance. Well, it isn't that simple. It kept my mom's skin smooth and bones strong, but in the end, those renegade hormones caused the cancer that killed her. (I am not against hormone therapy, but think it must be closely monitored.)

One proven fact is that food, especially fatty foods, heated up in the microwave in plastic containers, produces chemicals that poisons our bodies. We need to stop using plastic wrap to cover the foods you microwave, instead use glass, corning ware, or Pyrex to heat or re-heat. Empty out tv dinners and microwaveable foods from their plastic packaging and cook food in non-plastic containers.

Choosing the most helpful vitamins, minerals and supplements is trickier than you think. A balanced multi-vitamin and mineral supplement are good foundations, but often not adequate. As I said before, my mother's daily intake of eighty vitamins a day did not save her life, but she sure looked young when she died!

You can do everything right: eat the best food, think the best thoughts, exercise every day and still get cancer. There are genetic influences and viruses we don't know much about yet. Hopefully, someday there will be a vaccine for cancer and medicines that will keep it under control. Despite the barrage of conflicting health information, all we can do is take good care of our bodies the best way we know how. Hire a health coach, or find someone who can help you navigate the right dietary choices for your unique situation.

CHAPTER 18

What Now?

The last day of radiation was over! I was tired, weak and had continuous bowel drama, but I was happy to be alive. Now I could take it easy while my body recuperated from the year of stress. Or so I thought!

I had decided to move near Shanen in case I went down the cancer path again and needed her help. There was a 40% chance that the cancer might recur and the radiation had drained me of energy. I didn't have the strength in me to keep up with the yard or tackle all those little annoying things that can break down in an older house.

Moles were turning my backyard into their playground, my flower gardens were dying from neglect and my house was settling, revealing a crack in the ceiling of the living room. Every time I went outside to work in the yard, fire ants sent out the alert and hundreds came running to attack me. With every storm, I wondered if those giant pine trees in the backyard with their exposed shallow roots were going to fall down on my house.

To add to the stress, there was the parking problem in the cul-de-sac in front of my home. No one had enough room in their single car driveways for the two cars they had, so they parked their extra cars in the crowded turn-around. This caused a problem for the garbage trucks when they circled around to collect our trash, so they often didn't pick up the garbage. The rental house next door looked shabbier and shabbier as time went by and the landlord didn't care to keep it up. The house behind me had been turned over to the bank and was languishing in disrepair and weeds. Four years ago, my perfect house in a nice neighborhood had now begun to look bedraggled and was surrounded by bad company.

I could see that the neglected homes around me were not going to add to the value of my house and dealing with the garbage was a weekly aggravation. And those damn moles! I could not get rid of them and I would not resort to lethal traps. Someone told me to try shaving off pieces of Irish Spring soap and sprinkling the stinky soap shavings down their holes. That should take care of them, they assured me, but no, the smell just made me sick.

Then I bought some mole deterrent stakes to put in the ground which made beeping sounds every thirty seconds, supposedly like the sound of a wounded or distressed animal. This was to make the moles think there was danger nearby and cause them to run the other way. Sure, once the moles got the joke, they ignored the trills of the stakes while I kept looking for a phone that was ringing somewhere!

"Contact the King of the Moles," advised a friend who works with fairies and garden spirits. "Tell him to move his operation to the neighbor's yard." I did that, even explaining to the King that my neighbors never mowed their grass which would make life so much easier for his mole tribe. Nothing worked; they liked my yard best. My romance with my lovely home was over.

Since I was weak and unsure of my future, everything seemed overwhelming: the moles, the fire ants, the dying plants. My intuition said it was time to move, but my body said don't put me through THAT again. It was time to clean out the closets, go through a life-time of artwork, files of writing, boxes of mementos and hundreds of books, treasures and photos. I contacted a realtor and the fun of showing my house to prospective buyers began.

BC, or "before cancer," I had wanted to open an Air B & B and had begun the process. I was in a great location, living right down the road from the three most beautiful gardens and plantations in the world. And I had two extra bedrooms and a second bathroom. Also, I had remodeled my garage into an art studio space. It had taken me a year to change that blah garage into a comfortable art studio with its own cooling and heating system and ceiling fans. I painted the floors and created an abstract design on one of the walls. I never got to enjoy it; I prepared for one future and another one came my way instead.

The decision to sell my house came at a time when other upsetting things were happening. My wonderful terrier mix dog, George, had an accident three weeks after my diagnosis of cancer. One night at midnight, I saw he was in pain and rushed him to the emergency veterinarian hospital. Horrible news; he had broken his spine. A few days later he was operated on and couldn't move, didn't eat, and was drugged and pathetic. He stayed in the hospital for three weeks, barely recovering. I never knew what jump he had made that snapped his spine, since he bounded on and off the furniture constantly.

All I knew was that poor little George, the dog of my dreams, was now a cripple. I wondered if he would ever be able to use his back legs again. He was incontinent and had no control of his bowels. We had to express his bladder, massage him, ply him with pain pills and watch him every minute because he still thought he could jump around. I improvised a sling from a pair of my stretch pants and looped it under his tummy to hold up his back-end while we walked. Thankfully, his front legs still worked and his personality was intact, but my poor little boy was in such pitiful shape.

Along with Shanen's and Nick's help, I kept working on him, massaging his legs, moving them in circles, giving him CBD oil and cleaning up after him night and day. It seemed like he and I were both "poor things" wearing diapers—mine were Depends and his were made from doggy sanitary pads!

When it rains, it pours they say, for then, my beautiful Russian Blue cat, Momma Blue, developed a tumor in her intestines. In fact, one day I was taking notes from the vet on the results of a scan they did for her and then minutes after that conversation, I got a call from my doctor with the results of a scan they did on me. The two notes I wrote down were almost identical: inflamed lymph nodes, a tumor that needed to be excised, radiation and chemo to follow.

My cat was manifesting something so similar to what I was going through that I wondered if she were picking up on my disease and incorporating it into her body. Cancer isn't contagious, my vet reminded me when I told him my theory, but I do believe that pets will absorb the energy around them.

Many years ago, I read a book called *Dreaming Myself, Dreaming a Town,* by Susan Watkins, who explained that our pets will take on our maladies as a sacrifice to their beloved owners. I read other stories about people who swore that something like this had happened to them. In fact, I had had one such experience many years ago with my beloved black cat, Jazz.

At that time, I had a strange dream about Jazz rescuing me from dark underground tunnels. He was flying like Super-cat, while I trailed behind riding on his energy. He was saving me from an underworld space. Meanwhile, in real life, I was puzzled about his strange behavior of "telling" me something was wrong. He stretched himself out across the laps of my husband and me as we sat on the couch—something he had never done before. He wanted to be held like a baby and would sometimes get on my chest and position himself so he could put his face up against mine and look me in the eyes. Again, this was very unusual behavior for him. I knew something was up and took him to the vet in case he had a puncture wound that I couldn't see in his dense black fur. Nothing showed up.

At the time, I was suffering from bout after bout of bronchial problems, coughing so hard I saw stars which scared my daughters into thinking I might die. Doctors failed to help me. Suddenly, one morning I woke up to find Jazz, in pain. We rushed him to the vet and he died minutes later from an embolism bursting in his lungs. I don't know how all these events added up, but intuitively, I felt he had taken on my symptoms and sacrificed himself.

I believed something similar was happening with Momma Blue. My vet told me that her problems might be addressed if I took a chance on surgery, radiation and chemo for her. I was just beginning my cancer treatments and it was too much for me to tend to her needs, Georgie's needs and my own needs. I made a decision not to have the surgery for her. I decided to let nature take its course. She continued to live a happy life with me for over a year and a half. I believe we might not have had that year if I had started invasive medical treatment for her back then. It was a decision I did not make lightly.

I took Momma to the vet three times during that year to make sure she wasn't in pain and didn't have an infection. I was exhausted, cleaning up after my dog every few hours, going to a stream of doctor's appointments for myself and getting the house ready to sell.

Thankfully, my house sold quickly. The buyers were glad there was no Home Owners Association, loved the pine trees, didn't notice the popcorn ceilings and found my remodeled garage a perfect game room big enough for their pool table. As for my mole-riddled backyard, no problem—they were going to put in an in-ground pool. In one month, it was over. I reluctantly left my home, which was supposed to have been my forever home, and rented an apartment at an assisted living facility where I could transition to hospital care if needed. I did not know if the cancer would return and I wanted to be prepared.

I found it harder and harder to take care of George and his constant diapering needs, especially in my new apartment. I asked Shanen and my grandson, Jonathan, if they would keep Georgie for a while to relieve my stress. Luckily, they ended up falling in love with my sweet crippled boy and adopted him. He has lived with them for six months now and I know he is living the good life as a truly pampered pet. He has Jonathan to play with and my daughter treats him like a little prince. He is still crippled and wears diapers, but is able to run like a greyhound when there is a squirrel to chase!

At this point, Momma Blue had me all to herself. This aloof cat (a rescue ten years before and almost feral at the time) finally became an affectionate pet. She was happy it was just we two living in our little apartment. She slept a lot and allowed me to give her therapeutic massages, sometimes twice a day. She did what Jazz did when death had approached him; she climbed up on my chest, looked directly into my eyes and kissed my nose—my first kiss from her.

My gray velvet beauty would await her nightly massages impatiently, stamping her paws on the covers and meowing for me to hurry up! When I got settled in the bed, she would flop over against me, alerting me that this was time to begin her massage. I enjoyed kneading, stroking, scratching and giving compliments to her while she purred her approval. Her previous life as a feral cat, always on guard, was gone forever. She would roll over on her back and lift her front legs, one at a time, allowing me to massage her armpits! And to my surprise, I was able to rub each toe on every paw, giving her reflexology massages that any cat (or human) would die for. She had finally surrendered to love, coming a long way from the cat that didn't even want to be scratched under her chin.

As she dealt with her tumor problem and I dealt with mine, I wondered if once again I was seeing her do for me what I believed Jazz had done for me so many years before. Had she absorbed or taken on some of my illness, sacrificing her life? I asked her this one time telepathically and told her if the answer was "yes," for her to move from the bottom of the bed and lie down again next to my waist, stay a minute and then go back to her original spot. In less than a minute, she got up and did just that—not scientific proof, but good enough for me.

When I made the decision to let her go, I knew it was the right time. I called Shanen to meet me at the vet where I already had an appointment for Momma Blue's check-up. Suddenly that morning, I knew it was time to let her go. In the few days leading up to her appointment, she had stopped eating, greeting me and wanting her massages. I knew she was ready, but was I? I put her into her carrying case and for once she cooperated, not fighting me as she usually did. I called the vet and asked if my appointment time could be used for more than a check-up. What an intensely painful time it is bidding an animal farewell. Shanen and I cried like babies as we sat holding Momma Blue, loving on her and saying goodbye. I was so thankful for the sweet time the two of us had had together in my apartment where she didn't have to share me with George.

All through this difficult year of my animals having troubles, selling my house and moving, my cancer journey and losing Nick, it felt like I was balancing on a knife's edge of life and death. In December, three months after my last radiation treatment, I went to the cancer center at the hospital to have a scan to see how I was doing. A few days later, the results were ready and I made a second trip downtown for a physical exam with my surgeon and radiologist.

Dr. Gray and Dr. Cope were gathered with two nurses at the bottom of the exam table doing the physical exam. After looking at my scan results, they were thrilled to tell me that I was cancer free! I was so shocked that I couldn't take it in. I know I disappointed them with my blank stare while they had the most joyful expressions on their faces, relieved they got to share some good news with a patient. "You are *cancer-free*!" they repeated as if I hadn't heard them the first time.

I walked out of the cancer center into the dazzling December afternoon's sunlight. I was still in shock and drove home without feeling anything. I had believed I was going to die of cancer, that the cancer had spread and metastasized (as it had in my lymph node). But now I had to switch my mindset to a different channel. I had prepared for my death, arranged for the sale of my house, euthanized my cat, packed up hundreds of boxes and moved carload after carload of possessions to an assisted living facility—and now I wasn't going to die, I was going to live!

Part Three

CHAPTER 19

The Boogie Man Under the Bed

I've had several intense, life-changing dreams in my past. One that heralded a new chapter in my healing journey is this dream, which I entitled, "The Telling." It provided me the opportunity to speak my truth and have a witness. Here is the dream:

I am in my bedroom bed when grandpa comes in and falls on top of me. He is whispering sweet nothings in my ear pretending to be confused as to who I am. I am fighting him off me, yelling and struggling under the weight of him. He is frightened by my forcefulness. Nicole Brown Simpson (the murdered wife of O.J. Simpson) is standing off to the side and is my witness. I begin to drum on a little hand drum. I am letting the drum tell the tale. I want everyone to know I will no longer be a victim. I awake and find myself lying on my stomach and patting the mattress as if I am playing a drum.

An unexpected outcome of this dream was that after having it, I no longer awoke with my arms feeling paralyzed. For decades, I would awaken many mornings to find my entire arms, from shoulders to hands, numb. I sleep on my back, so it wasn't because of the position of my body while I slept. To remedy the situation, I would scoot myself to sitting upright, lean against the headboard and flop my limp arms around to bring life back into them. In a minute or two, energy flooded back into my arms and I would go on with my morning routine. I never had a second thought about whether this was normal or not. I never told anyone—not even a doctor—about this. After the drumming dream, the strange affliction with my paralyzed arms disappeared.

Weird things like this happened to me throughout my life, but I didn't know they were unusual. It was normal to keep things buried from conscious awareness. As a family, we kept our secrets in sealed containers and never compared notes. Life went on, as if it were normal to have a raging drunk urinating in the front yard or passed out and carried home by his bar buddies.

One time grandpa had the dt's (delirious tremors) and grandma told me not to go near the bedroom door because grandpa had his rifle loaded and might shoot at his "demons" and inadvertently shoot me. I nodded that I understood the warning and went to the kitchen for some chips and a soft drink. I turned on *Lassie* and watched Timmy tell Lassie to go get Grandpa as my grandpa raged and cursed those demons attacking him in his bedroom. I took the long way to the bathroom just in case bullets started flying. I was an adult before I realized this drama was not a normal family night.

I loved the family television sitcoms where things were normal—nothing dark or scary ever happened. I have heard stories from many adults who had rocky childhoods saying that they also loved happy shows like *Father Knows Best.* I wanted so much to be the youngest daughter nicknamed "Kitten" and I wanted the actor Robert Young to be my real dad. I didn't see much of my father who lived across town and was caught up in his business success and new family. He had no idea of what was going on in the home where I lived with my grandparents.

Later in life, I asked some girlfriends I grew up with if it was common knowledge that my grandfather was the village drunk. They said no. It was lucky for me that their parents let them come over to play with me and thankfully I never felt ostracized. As an adult, I ran into my old Campfire group leader who knew me as a child from nine to thirteen years old. In a short chat about those days, she surprised me by saying, "Everyone was worried about you!"

That my grandpa was a pedophile didn't register with me for a long time. I remember getting an uncomfortable feeling in my stomach as a teen when he showed an inordinate interest in a pretty neighbor girl who was maturing into a teen. When he started asking me questions about her, it gave me the chills.

The fact that my mother confessed to me his abuse of her when I was a young adult always made me feel sorry for her, not ever thinking about myself. Through her, I learned the story of how our family (my grandparents and their three children: my mother and two uncles) snuck out of town one night, forced to leave their home and comfortable lives in Kentucky. They moved to Ohio in order for Grandpa to escape an enraged father who was after him—intent on killing him for "messing" with his daughter. That was Kentucky justice in the 1930's.

My grandparents and their three children went from riches to rags—from my grandfather having money and owning a lumberyard business in Berea, Kentucky, to moving to a run-down farm that his sister owned in Ohio. Grandpa was not a family man, but he was a diligent worker and there was always food on the table. Unfortunately, at that table my uncles and mom, as children, would be cursed and smacked around. Alcohol, abuse, and the Great Depression were all factors in their lives. Grandpa had mellowed somewhat by the time I lived with him, never cursing or beating me as he had my mother and uncles.

I knew enough about my grandfather's childhood to know it was no picnic. He quit school and went to work picking up coal on railroad tracks at eight years old. He was in the Navy for a brief period and there began his drinking and womanizing career. He met and married an innocent farm girl, who had never been on a date. My grandma quickly found out that her husband was an angry and mean alcoholic who made life hell for her and their children.

Generation after generation, we were a family caught up in the dynamics and denial of alcohol and abuse, living in a trance of dysfunction. Back in those days, there wasn't any information about how to break the chains of addiction; all the self-help groups were not yet available. We staggered on in our dysfunctional lives doing the best we could, completely ignorant of how alcohol affected families.

For me, trying to put the pieces together of my puzzling childhood was a life-long struggle. I knew that alcoholism took a terrible toll on all of us. My body knew the truth that something wasn't right—this wasn't the way life was supposed to be. When my grandfather asked me to marry him, I laughed it off and then went into my bedroom and hid. I felt like I was in a Tennessee Williams' play—something that felt depraved, mythic and dark, and definitely not like *Father Knows Best*.

I was robbed of safety, protection, self-worth and innocence. I have had to ask my body to forgive me for years of neglect and denial. I have had to acknowledge that my life's shame and confusion kept me from feeling my true worth and achieving my dreams. I had to expend a lot of energy evading the big bad wolf and it has taken me years to trade in my red hooded cloak of victimization.

I graduated with honors from high school and entered the college world where I did not feel comfortable. I had the brains and looked the part of a pretty confident co-ed, but dating was overwhelming to me. I did not approve of that college's sorority system which banned Jews and Blacks. I refused the invitation; that kind of mentality was not for me. Other than that, I didn't know who I was or what I wanted to do in life. I was overwhelmed by male attention and freaked out at the sexual overtures I was experiencing when dating. I had what was then called a nervous breakdown, quit college and went home to escape a life that I wasn't prepared for.

I couldn't find or keep a job. I had no career goals or aspirations except one—to meet my prince and be whisked away to a sweet home with a picket fence. I met a lot of toads and some really nice guys whose value I did not recognize at the time. I was not the princess I portrayed myself to be to them. If they only knew that I felt like a toad myself.

I had many breakdowns including one that put me in bed in my grandparent's attic for a year of self-isolation. This was all before antidepressants were on the market which could have changed my life. I stayed in that bed upstairs in the attic day after day because I could not get up and be in the world. In my mind, I was bad, ugly, weak and powerless. I developed what I believe was BDD—Body Dysmorphic Disorder (this was before it was a diagnosis). That part of my life is hard to think about because it was so painful. I wasted many years of my youth hiding from life. I knew I had to change, get on the right track and have a life. I just didn't know where that track was.

During my twenties, I lived in New York City, Virginia Beach, Virginia; Dayton, Ohio; Laguna Beach, California; Homestead, Florida and back to Dayton many times in between. Changing locations did not solve my problems, for wherever I moved, there I was. My hormones and my extreme moods always caught up with me. I was running from all of it: my past, my shame, my perceived failures. Watching my friends who were graduating, beginning careers, getting married and starting families made me feel even more flawed. I panicked and married on impulse and to who else—but an alcoholic whose name was the same as my grandpa's! That marriage was short-lived and thankfully, with no children involved.

I saw a few therapists whenever I could afford to and went to sexual survivor support groups. I tried hypnotherapy, rebirthing, talk therapy, pounded a pillow with my fists, screamed, cried and kept trying to find peace and healing. I studied my dreams, developed some insights about my family and became interested in spirituality.

I was growing up in spite of myself. Maturity was finally helping me to have a somewhat normal life as I continued trying to put the pieces of the puzzle together. Just who was crazy in this family of mine? Was it me or had I soaked up all the craziness around me?

Several therapists I went to praised me by saying I was doing pretty well with my life considering my past. I have since learned that almost all survivors of childhood molestation carry the shame of the crime, while the perpetrators and the "innocent on-lookers" go free of retribution and rarely have any awareness of or guilt about what is going on.

I went back and forth from temporary office jobs, working as a waitress, cleaning houses, and taking college classes when time allowed and I felt up to it. I tried to find a path and start a career. I was a preschool teacher with three and four-year old children, but quickly found I didn't have the patience for that. Next, I tried working with abused children in foster care. I was part of a therapy department in what they used to call an orphanage. I wasn't a bona fide social worker, but acted as an assistant in play therapy, testing and writing reports on how the children were doing within their foster families. I was finding I had some skills in this arena and began feeling better about myself. I also found out that social workers have a limited career, since the emotional drain on them is intense. I wasn't able to last too long in this stressful field, either.

About this time, I met Dave, a therapist in training, who gave me a break on expensive therapy sessions called re-parenting. He introduced me to a healing dynamic called cathecting or Cathexis, pioneered by Jacqui Schiff (author of the book, *All My Children*). Dave and his wife Marilyn re-parented me with some new messages about life. I actually rewrote my birth scene from what I knew of my mother's birth stories, only this time I had a good safe delivery. I was naked and greased up with coconut oil and squeezed out easily from between two bean bag chairs into the arms of my "father", played by Dave, who welcomed me into the world.

Then I was regressed and re-experienced some very young ages where I received loving messages from my new mother and father as played by Dave and Marilyn. I remember crawling around and deciding to make a break for freedom. I gleefully began to escape up the stairs to push my limits. My "father" stopped me and in a gentle way showed me that I would not be punished for normal behavior like that of testing my limits. This "do over" gave me a sense of security I hadn't had before.

Things were definitely improving for me. The

cathecting therapy healed something inside me and I was developing confidence. I had stopped bouncing back and forth from living at my grandparent's house to my father's home and was living in my own cozy mobile home. I was taking college classes and excelling in art. I joined a pottery cooperative and fell in love with clay. I was having successes at work, art, and was also doing some freelance work as a magician's assistant. It was during this time that I met a gentle man with a good heart who seemed like a perfect fit for the role of my prince. He was a Captain in the Air Force and worked at Wright Patterson Air Force Base as a scientist in the laser laboratory. It was the time to try marriage again and I felt this time I had made a good choice. After a year of dating, we married.

We bought a house with more than just a white picket fence; we also had a vegetable garden, fruit trees, a rose garden, a magical wooded glade and a dog. We were not planning to have any children, but during a blizzard we got pregnant and our daughter arrived nine months later as did many other "blizzard babies." So many babies arrived the night of my labor that a young intern was rounded up from the hospital's cafeteria to help the one and only doctor on ward that night.

Of course, it was the full moon and all seven women from my Lamaze class were lined up in the halls moaning and groaning. I was having back labor and going "natural." I was screaming, "I've changed my mind! Give me that epidural!" They wouldn't, saying, "Too late now!" We were in a bad way, my daughter and me. She wasn't able to make her way down the birth canal positioned backwards, so every contraction pushed her against my spinal cord instead of out the exit door. She was stuck, and the doctor began talking about a C-section. Finally, she arrived, popping out so fast the doctor almost dropped her. She was a beautiful shade of blue. The nurses took her away from me and I did not see her until the next day. It was a most brutal and primitive experience for us both.

I was very happy to be a mother, but hadn't counted on a baby with colic. It was hard to get up three and four times a night to nurse and spend the day rocking a screaming baby in pain. My husband was often out of town for his job and I had no babysitters I could trust with a newborn. As a mother, I felt like I would go crazy that first winter. The stress was so bad that I ended up with a heart arrhythmia.

In a couple years, our infant daughter turned into a toddler and I thankfully quit breastfeeding since she was cutting her front teeth on my nipples. One day, I felt an overwhelming need to get back into my art and express what I had been through. I asked for a full day to go into my studio and create. My husband cooperated and in a state of frenzy and happiness, I created sixteen collages that illustrated all the changes and challenges I was going through. Art has saved my sanity many times.

In fact, art and writing are the ways I process my life. They help me understand what is going on. The collages came pouring out of me with subjects on childbirth, my childhood, motherhood, my identity and spontaneous themes I didn't know were wanting expression. One of the collages featured a photograph of my grandfather and me when I was about four years old. I put a piece of netting over it and under the photo I glued my childhood skate key. There were other symbolic items glued onto the canvas that I didn't understand at the time. Not long after I completed this collage, I picked it up and took it to the trash can and threw it away. There was something I did not want to look at in that collage. Luckily, I took a photo of it before I destroyed it and was later able to discern what the collage was telling me.

I had begun to write some articles for our newspaper in Dayton, Ohio before I had my baby, so I continued doing interviews, often taking her with me. I was trying to hold onto bits and pieces of myself. I didn't want to drown in diapers and baby food. I had no idea that motherhood could change you into something that didn't come close to who you were up until then. I wanted to keep as much of myself that I could and that involved books. I remember reading Marilyn French's book *The Women's Room* on my lap while sitting on the toilet and nursing my baby all at the same time. I discovered that with children comes multi-tasking.

I was determined not to forgo my reading, dancing, yoga, women's group or sense of self because I was now a mother. I didn't know that surrender was part of the deal. As much as I loved being a mother, I was not a superwoman. I look back and know I was so needing help. Just the fact that I had not had a full night's sleep for over a year made me nutty. My husband challenged me by saying, "What's the matter with you? Look at all these women who have more than one child. They are doing fine." I later found out that was rarely true. Our marriage began breaking down when I saw he couldn't extend a hand to me when I felt like I was drowning.

I enjoyed the success of writing for the newspaper and for local trade magazines. I created art with my little girl and enjoyed summer visits from my step-daughter who lived in Texas with her mom and brother. I tried to be a good wife, good mother, social planner, sexual playmate and fun person, but I was going crazy. I was a child of divorce and determined not to do that to my daughter. I wanted to stay the course and not allow myself to go to bed and pull the covers over my head.

Unfortunately, my mom moved back home to Dayton from her beloved New York City. My mother wanted to become a grandmother so badly *and* she wanted to become the mother of my daughter, bumping me out of the way. She judged me a terrible mother and made my life hell for the next eighteen years. The tension and disagreements were terrible between us. I had raging episodes that scared everybody, including me. I was angry at my mother, upset with my husband and still dealing with bouts of depression.

My marriage was a constant source of irritation. I wanted authenticity. I wanted communication. I wanted my husband to have my back in my war with my mother who was determined to undermine my relationship with my daughter. He did not know how to give me any kind of emotional support but to tell me he loved me. Communication at a deep level was not his thing and I was starved for it. I was not easy to live with and had many childhood issues still boiling beneath the surface. Ever since my daughter turned four, I had been having disturbing dreams about sexual abuse. I was tormented, and my husband's advice was to go out and jog.

I begged him to read one slim book I found on the subject of how to support a loved one who was dealing with abuse. I saw the book lay on his bedside table buried under articles and newspapers for months. I asked him a few times if he would read it and then gave up, realizing that what I wanted from him, he just couldn't give to me.

The following dream alerted me that I had better leave the marriage before it killed me:

> *I am in a coffin, lying there alive with the lid open. My husband is standing next to it with a hammer and nails ready to hammer the coffin lid shut. I wake up with the chills. I know I have to face the fact that he is going to do something to me that will suffocate me.*

I woke up wondering if some people stay in a marriage that is slowly killing them rather than face the dread, the finality, the "failure" of divorce. There is suffering either way. This dream brought the danger of staying in my marriage front and center. I wanted to live, so I prepared to go.

After twenty years of good times and struggles, we ended the marriage. Rochelle was married by then and Shanen was off to college. I knew I must divorce, even if leaving the familiar feathered nest created some anxiety. I wish I could say I sailed through the divorce, but no— it was one of the most painful things I have ever done. Because there was much love between my husband and me, it was gut-wrenching to part ways. I cried my way through it. Oh, the price of freedom. I dreamt about him for years and felt we were still married even though we both had found other partners.

CHAPTER 20

Together Again

A year after my divorce, I met a handsome man named Nick at a divorce support group meeting. We sat next to each other, talked easily, and it felt natural to invite him over to my house to watch a television show featuring presentations on various religions. We found we shared a deep interest in spiritual growth. We had many talks about his Catholic upbringing and the wonderful breakthrough he had had from a Catholic program called Cursillo.

Nick wanted to show me his favorite place: Charleston, South Carolina, where his work had taken him in the past. We took a trip to the Holy City during the prime time of spring when an international art festival called Spoleto is in full bloom there. I fell in love with the Lowcountry: the culture, the art, the beauty, the ocean, just as Nick had predicted I would.

There was no staying in Dayton after that visit! Nick and I packed up and moved with all the belongings we could pack into a U-Haul and our two dogs, to South Carolina. I didn't know what I would do once I got there, but surely my art career was a fit for such an arty city. And it was. I began teaching all kinds of art classes to kids and adults at a fantastic art center. I wrote a play and had it produced with the support of an art grant and made a documentary film about women and their feelings regarding their bodies, called *The Breast Dialogues*. I exhibited my art and Nick and I found a church we liked.

I was living my dream in Charleston, but sadly, my dear Nick struggled to find his niche. I was carrying the financial load, which was hard on our relationship. Our partnership finally broke down and we ended up living separately and finally, after a while, called it quits. It was hard to see him out dating, especially since I had no love interest on the horizon. I missed him and my close connection with his mother and daughter. It felt like another divorce.

I decided I needed a new location, since I was running into Nick constantly—even at midnight in Walmart's produce department! I knew wherever I went—to an art festival, a play, a music venue, the supermarket, there would be Nick. I was unhappy, so I decided to move to the Asheville area where I had a few friends. Once there, I began to develop a life; finding a church, some artistic friends, classes to take and teach, but then it snowed! I do not like snow. It is one of the reasons I loved the Charleston area—a light snow flurry once every few winters is enough for me.

Not only did it snow in Asheville, but it was such a heavy snow that it kept me marooned in my home for five days. Although the mountains were lovely, the people were great, the town charming, and the art and music festivals extraordinary, I didn't want to live anywhere there was snow.

That's when my dad called me and asked me to come back to Dayton. He wasn't doing well physically and neither was my mom. I felt a daughterly obligation to go, plus I was grieving the breakup with Nick and I was feeling unsettled about Asheville. Once again, I moved my stuff in a U-Haul truck and returned to Dayton to start another chapter.

I set up housekeeping in a cute ranch-style house and reconnected with friends and family there. I knew I had a job to do, which was to help my parents, who were going downhill at the same time. They hadn't been married to each other for decades, but still had a telephone contact relationship. I went from checking in on my dad, at his home where he lived alone since my stepmom had died a few years before, to checking in on my mom where she lived in an apartment building which housed seniors.

It was hell dealing with both of them day after day. My father had to be in absolute control. He was too far gone mentally to make good decisions, but he insisted on managing his life—he would have it no other way. I could not wrestle control away from him even though it would have been in his best interest. I had him evaluated and since he knew the date, his name and the President's name, I could not prove his incompetence to the law. He was out of control, and still driving—too fast and too recklessly.

Dad was being scammed by some former employees; one of whom wanted him to give her a million dollars so she could start a car wash that would employ teenagers.

She got quite a bit of money out of him before he was too sick to read her letters. His mailbox was full of thank you letters and please send more money letters from various "so called" non-profits. I showed him my research that proved his donations were going directly into the pockets of CEO's of the businesses. This enraged him, as he believed in their validity and resented me for showing him the evidence.

My father was profoundly deaf, but refused to get a hearing aid except to order a cheap one from a magazine which squealed non-stop. When he had a hernia repaired, he refused to go back for the follow-up appointment. Dad's partial plate didn't fit right, so he played "dentist" and used a metal file to file it down, destroying it. And there were other problems.

His constant battle with the neighbors about property issues was a daily drama. The neighbors had their fill of his craziness and were going to take legal recourse. I called and persuaded them to have mercy on my dad, explaining he had nothing to do all day, so writing letters to them and calling the authorities regarding the dispute kept his mind active. I admired his attempts to be engaged with life even though he was driving me nuts. He refused up to the very end of his life to go to a care facility. His life ended at age 94 after breaking his hip and a bout with pneumonia.

My mother was as strong-willed as ever, too. She wanted to stay in control of her finances, medical treatment and all decisions concerning her life. Her doctor was charmed by her and prescribed whatever she asked him to—that's why she liked him so much, plus the fact he played the didgeridoo in his office. She wanted to manage her affairs and did a pretty good job doing so. My job was to cook meals, visit, spend some overnights, take her out when she was up to it and try to be "the good daughter." Because of her traumatic childhood, Mom was never a good parent to me, but I did what I could to keep things peaceful between us. Sadly, we never had the closure we both needed.

In 2013, my mom died in the spring, after four years of suffering from cancer. My dad followed her a few months later in September. They both died with their eyes wide open, looking for their next adventure. I have a photo of them from the early days of their marriage looking like Bonnie and Clyde, standing in front of their 1940's Ford. Even though they were only married seven years before divorcing, I could see how the wild streaks of their youth attracted each other.

After my mom died and was cremated, and my dad had a soldier's burial a few months later, my daughterly duty was done. I was exhausted. I couldn't wait to get back to the place I loved, beautiful South Carolina. I packed up my belongings once again and found an apartment for me and my dog, called old friends and looked around to see what was in store for me in this chapter of my life.

One day, I was standing alone in the middle of Marion Square in downtown Charleston, looking around at the dwindling crowd after a Thanksgiving parade. My girlfriend had abandoned me to go talk to her friends when someone came up behind me and grabbed me in a big bear hug. It was Nick! He was downtown for the parade and had been sitting at an outdoor table with his girlfriend, when she pointed me out to him. We hadn't seen each other in five years. We were so happy that we couldn't stop talking and catching up. That poor girlfriend was totally forgotten, knowing there was an instant connection between Nick and me and it was over for her.

Nick and I took up where we left off, but this time older and wiser. We were both orphans now, since his delightful mother, Dot, had died while I was in Dayton. Our lives were coasting along with the simple things in life: church, friends, family, pets, volunteering at the animal shelter and a few day trips to nearby towns when Nick's health began to deteriorate at a rapid pace and I got cancer. Even though we both had health problems, we were thankful to be living in such a beautiful place and to have each other.

CHAPTER 21

Standing in the Paradox

Thanks to that onion jamming itself under my gas pedal, I was warned that something was coming down the pike. Without that warning, my journey would have been so much more terrifying.

The word onion is derived from *"unio,"* meaning unity. Ancient Egyptians viewed the many layers of the onion as a symbol for eternity. To them, it represented the multi-layers of reality and the balance between all elements.

On the negative side, the onion represents tears, memories, disguises, evil spirits and jealousy. In India, an onion is hung on the wall near a sick person to absorb the illness; not a bad idea considering the onion's antibacterial quality. One component of the onion's chemistry, allicin, is used for repairing skin scars. Homemade brews of boiled honey and onions have been used for generations as a cough tonic or poultice.

It's a pretty amazing plant (with over one hundred varieties) which is currently being researched for its healing potential for cancer and other diseases. Onions also contain quercetin, which has shown to slow down cancer cell growth. Eating onions, raw or cooked, supplies the body with some protection against heart attacks, pancreatic cancer, stomach cancer, diabetes and endometrial cancer. These findings are from various studies done by universities all over the world.

My own hospital, MUSC (Medical University of South Carolina), analyzed data from the National Health and Nutrition Examination Survey and found perimenopausal and postmenopausal women who ate onions every day had a five percent density improvement in their bones. Not much difference, but every little bit helps women on the edge!

I like the metaphor of the onion because I have had to peel away many layers to get to the core of my life. I did it through life experiences, therapy, dream work, reading inspiring books, spiritual growth, honest relationships and supportive friendships. I meditated, studied symbols, journaled, went from therapist to therapist and staggered on at times in the depths of depression. No matter what twist or turn my life took, I had an inner "memo" from my spirit that I was worth it and deserved a healthy whole life. Inside all those layers of drama and trauma, there was an inner peace to be found.

When I was diagnosed with cancer of the vagina, there was a message from my body that I could not deny. My body was speaking to me as it always had—in the only way it knew how—with symptoms. My understanding of these symptoms was the final piece of the puzzle.

I was molested by someone I loved. I didn't want to accept it and my therapists couldn't push me to deal with the crime until I was ready. I buried it deep in my psyche, but my body brought it to the surface time and again in physical problems.

I didn't want to give up the images of my childhood that I held dear. I didn't want to give up my love for my grandfather. For a long time, I didn't know how to stand in the paradox of loving and hating my grandfather at the same time. I could mourn that no one "saved me" or "had my back." Those adults surrounding me were collectively unconscious and/or totally immersed in their own dramas. I am angry at being robbed of innocence and having to spend so many distressing years damaged, lost and searching for the truth. But I can feel triumphant for having empowered myself with seeking help, doing the painful inner work and persevering to achieve a reasonably happy life.

There is still a big piece I am working on now—forgiveness. I regret the years I lived crippled by incest. I now forgive myself for doing the only thing I could do at the time. Not the best thing, but the *only* thing—I went unconscious, too.

Cancer taking over my female parts certainly got my attention. I now talk to my vagina in the most comforting and loving way, saying: you do not have to carry this burden anymore. I thank my lymph system for the excellent job it did for me. I tell my body how much I appreciate it as I shower and wash each part. I take long baths by candle light to luxuriate with my body in a sensual way. Besides feeling good, this calibrates my body with my mind and soul.

Sharing my story in the black and white print of this

book has been difficult at times, but I know there is healing through expression instead of suppression—that leads to depression. People often say they are thankful that cancer came into their lives and for the lessons they learned—mostly to live in the present and be thankful for each day that is given.

I learned that I could not escape from my past—it was embedded in my body. I learned to listen to my symptoms as presented by cancer. It wasn't easy. I didn't like it. I don't want to do it again even though it (the learning) was the gift of the cancer.

I have been cancer-free for over one year, according to a recent PET scan that indicated all is well. For now, I want to enjoy life even though we are in the midst of a pandemic and have just experienced the most disturbing and contentious presidential election in the history of our country. Having good health makes everything in life easier.

Author Kat Duff, who suffered from devastating chronic fatigue syndrome for years, ends her book, *Alchemy of Illness*, this way: "I hope I do not forget when I get well."

I don't want to forget either. So I tell myself to stay awake, pay attention, listen carefully to what the world around you brings your way. All of Life is talking to you—there is guidance everywhere waiting to be acknowledged—especially the moments that knock you off your feet. That is the main message of this book. Cancer revealed a lie that impacted my whole life. I say thank you to that onion for helping me accept my journey with cancer.

The search for the truth is not easy, but it is possible to know ourselves as we are in essence: the good parts and the "bad," the ugly and the beautiful, the profane and the sacred. The truth will set you free.

Finis

Postscript:

Cancer is a terrible disease; painful, heartbreaking, and for many, a disease that leads to death. My account is about my personal journey that involved looking at my past, following my intuition, examining dreams and symbols for clues, researching, reflecting and meditating. At a different point in my life, I might have made different choices and had a totally different experience. I am merely sharing what happened to me. It is my hope that I have presented you with some options for your journey.

Please know, dear reader, I do not think *all* cancers come from unresolved childhood issues or that all accidents have hidden motivations. I bring these things to light for your consideration.

Part Four

CHAPTER 22
Meditation

Meditation certainly helped me through the Year of the Onion. I want to encourage anyone going through a life-threatening illness to consider this practice. It seems to me that meditation is often described as detailed, esoteric and must be done in a certain way to get results. I want to reassure the reader that this is not necessarily true. Meditation does *not* have to be difficult or complicated. The problem for most of us is that our monkey minds want to sabotage the experience because our ego wants to run the show. There we sit, lie or walk, trying to become still, as our thoughts buzz around in our heads like a swarm of annoying mosquitoes. Frustrated, we often give up as stillness eludes us. We might even feel like failures.

Meditation, the word itself, summons up mystery, metaphysics and mysticism. However, it is a simple process that aligns one with their inner Spirit. The only thing in the way is the ego, which makes it difficult to obtain an empty mind. And that is the secret to meditation. Eliminating the ego makes us a transparency for the Light to shine through.

It is said that prayer is talking to God and meditation is listening to God. *All right, God, I will listen.* I affirm, as the Bible advises, to "Be still and know that I am God." *Here I am, still as a mouse, quiet and patient.* The minutes tick by as I listen. *Oh no, here they come, those distracting thoughts again: the shopping list, the to-do list, the problems of the day, life's dramas, the itch on my nose, a cramp in my toes and my stomach is growling. What's for dinner?* That's it—I tried, I showed up, I'm willing, and what did I get? Frustration!

I know that frustration well. I decided at various points in my life to pursue meditation using mantras (chants), yantras (visual aids), breathing techniques, affirmations and rituals to help me concentrate. I stared for hours at a candle flame as my focusing tool. I lit incense, chanted Om, fasted, prayed and locked my legs in the lotus position and stood on my head (yes, both at the same time). All I got were little spaces of "no mind" flickering by, but no big explosions of light. I wanted to be knocked off my ass like Saint Paul was knocked off his donkey on his journey to Damascus.

As a young adult, I studied Hatha Yoga and loved moving my body, holding it in asanas or postures and breathing in rhythm to the movements. Relaxing into the corpse pose, flat on the floor like a dead body at the yoga session's end, gave me the opportunity to tune into each part of my body and send it love, health and light. The deep breathing techniques changed my brain waves, but rarely did I achieve the no-mind state of true meditation. With the arrival of cancer, you'd better believe I decided to try harder! I can now say I have reached a level of meditation that is rewarding because I have found a way that works for me.

In meditation, we are not trying to do anything, achieve anything, go anywhere, collect merits or cultivate magical powers so we can find parking places downtown. Meditation is letting go of everything: our destinies, our world, our logic, our desires, our identities, our monkey minds—it all must go to make space for the stillness.

It is very hard for the ego to be pushed out of the way. The struggle with the ego leads many people to give up on meditation. What you have to give up on is YOU (your ego) being in control. Instead of thinking how difficult meditation can be, here's a way to think of it in a positive manner: Meditation is a sacred time; a sweet appointment to go within to meet with the Over Soul (Inner Self, God, Higher Power, Spirit, Creative Intelligence, Mother-Father-God, whatever you want to call it). That quiet time will manifest eventually in the peace that is the place of connection that you are seeking. I don't mean a connection between two separate entities, you and God, but an opening to make space for the God within you to blossom forth into your awareness of who you really are.

The many books on meditation, CD's, DVDs, and internet videos can be helpful or sometimes overly complicated. If the latter, you may be tempted to give up before you even start. Detailed illustrations of the chakras opening, the Kundalini rising, the Shakti and Shiva intertwining, dragons guarding the fortress gates in mandalas, mudras (holding your hands in sacred positions), postures (yoga), fasting, how to breathe from alternate nostrils—it's a little much for a beginner who just wants some peace of mind.

You can have a quick meditation anytime, anywhere, even waiting in the check-out line at the supermarket. You don't have to chant, breathe a certain way or even close your eyes. Just look at all those beautiful people around you: the cashier in her own little world of scanning groceries while she chats away with customers, the child in the cart in front of you making faces, the people coming in and out of the supermarket intent on their coupons and shopping lists. Become present in that moment and look at what is going on. It's all so humanly beautiful! Go within for a moment and feel gratitude and compassion—maybe even love—for the incredible human race.

Often, that awareness is enough for me to transcend the mundane material world and enter into a few blissful moments of no-mind—meditation. That's when my conscious mind stops processing and lets go of control. Yes, even a few seconds of awareness and surrender at the supermarket can bring a feeling of Oneness.

You will know that you are making progress with meditation when someone cuts you off in traffic and you just smile and bless them on their journey. Meditation takes you off the hamster wheel. Stop thinking, analyzing, worrying, distracting, procrastinating and judging for just a few minutes! Your spirit yearns to be filled with peace and sanity.

Through meditation, you will start to be able to see through the "mirror darkly" of the projection of everyday life. Dramas lessen, peace ensues, and here comes the drum roll—you and I are made for this! It is a secret that is revealed in a very detailed way in the Hindu scriptures and also in the symbolic allegories and parables in the Bible.

We are designed to become One with whatever you want to call it—Spirit, Soul, the Oversoul, Creative Intelligence, Mother-Father God. In Psalm Twenty-three, we are asked to "lie down in green pastures beside the still water" so our souls can be restored. How beautiful an invitation is that?

At the end of his life, Sir Francis Crick, of the DNA discovery fame, was researching the claustrum part of the brain announcing he had discovered the "seat of the soul." This, Crick said, was the most exciting discovery of his life! As a contemporary scientist, he thought he had discovered something new, but ancients mystics have written much about the seat of the soul.

Nestled snugly in the center of the brain are the higher centers (chakras) or light transformers, just waiting to be activated. The claustrum, septum pellucidum, hypothalamus, pineal and pituitary, besides their regular jobs, are also receivers of energy. They hold the secret of enlightenment (seeing the light, being filled with light) for they contain the "secret" (secretions) that are needed to spark the movement of energy from our lower chakras up to our higher chakras. When the energy reaches the chakra at the top of your head, transcendence from the material and mundane world to the spiritual is then experienced and we are in the Light (enlightened).

Transcendence is a state of bliss, enlightenment and expansion. When you realize you are One with all that is, it eliminates the desire to be angry with anyone. That is you whom you are pointing your finger at! Enlightenment is an experience that wakes us up from the hypnotized state we are in most of the time and allows us to see the whole picture.

Martin Luther King, Jr. described it in his speeches as going "to the mountain top." Author William James called it cosmic consciousness and mystic Joel Goldsmith referred to it as the realization of oneness. I think Walt Whitman described the experience quite beautifully in his epic poem, *Leaves of Grass*, where he acknowledges oneness with everything.

All cultures have references to the "shining skull" experience. We see the glow of halos illustrated in some Bibles around the heads of Jesus, Mary, his disciples and angelic beings. I have an old Bible in which the artist depicts the entire aura as a light outlining their bodies.

The awareness and the connection of your soul with God, or the Oversoul, is your destiny. We are told in sacred scriptures and in *A Course in Miracles* that we will all experience the awakening eventually. The timing is different for everyone. When you do take that journey and reach enlightenment, your world will change. You will see the life and the light in everyone and everything. There will no longer be anything to forgive. You will become aglow because you are now transparent. People will see and feel that light and your countenance will be a blessing to all.

The rising of the energy that activates the chakras is compared to a serpent wiggling its way from the bottom of your spine to the top of the head. Its energetic movement is called the rising of the Kundalini. It has a cleansing action on each of your centers as it travels up your spine. It is the Bible's allegorical "Jacob's ladder."

The ancient caduceus symbol seen on many medical emblems is the staff (the spine) with two serpents criss-crossing over each other from the bottom of the staff to the top. That is the kundalini as it activates the chakras. At the top of the symbol are two wings open like angel's wings, indicating the end of the journey where the kundalini transmutes from the body (serpent) to a higher state of mind.

Now that I have explained this physical event, I advise you not to worry about it. Although there are practices (especially in yoga) that educate and prepare a person for the rising of the kundalini, they may or may not be helpful to you. Ascetics, yogis, saints, gurus and devotees work at it full time in terms of celibacy, purification exercises, prayers, studies, service, rituals and fasting, but for most seekers, I don't believe we have to make it such an intensive experience.

Here's a guided imagery script that helps me meditate. I have done it so many times it is second nature. It moves me from my ordinary monkey mind to a peaceful place of stillness.

It's a lovely summer's day that finds me standing by a pond of clear water surrounded by trees. I throw in a small stone and watch the ripples of concentric circles expand out. The rings in the pond from the stone represent my intention to clear my mind of all thoughts. Those widening circles on the water represent my consciousness expanding and pushing my thoughts away further and further until they disappear. I throw in stone after stone—as many as I need to—until I have settled into a quiet mental state. Then, I pick up a rock (about the size of a grapefruit) and throw it into the center of the pond. It lands with a big plop. I watch that heavy rock sink slowly to the bottom of the pond. I suggest to myself that I, too, am going deeper and deeper, as I sink into my inner self. The rock gently comes to rest on the sandy bottom of the pond. My awareness has made the journey down deep, too. I am a rock with no thoughts. I wait. There is nothing to wait for. I listen. There is no sound. Only stillness. I experience the stillness. My mind is empty. I am in a meditative state.

Sometimes it lasts for a few minutes, sometimes for a half hour. When I come back to myself, I might feel a little sedated and take a minute to sense I am back in my body before I get up and drive somewhere.

Do I get that big lighting strike of the shining skull explosion? No, not yet. I just know my meditation is enough for now to stop the ego's grasp. I let expectations go and do not worry about whether this is "true meditation," or if I am doing it "right." I do not want to judge myself or compare my experience with others.

You will be surprised how the fruits of meditation show up in your life. They may be so subtle you don't see them at first. Maybe your blood pressure will normalize. Maybe your temper won't flare up as often. Maybe your addictions to shopping or drinking will lessen. As you include meditation practice into your daily life, you will notice changes that will make your effort worthwhile. Eventually, you will crave this time of delicious peace.

Experiment and find out what works for you. If you need something more than my style of visualization, consider other techniques like breathing exercises, movement (dance, yoga), sound (music, chants, drumming), inspirational poetry (Rumi, Hafiz), guided imagery or any rituals that may help you focus.

There are simple how-to books on meditation (Lawrence Leshan's: *How to Meditate)* and esoteric classics like *The Secret of the Golden Flower,* a translation of the ancient Chinese text of Tao, by scholar Richard Wilhelm. Deepak Chopra has all kinds of resources on meditation and the evolution of the spirit. Yoga and meditation teachers have a variety of techniques to share. Take some time and explore what fits for you.

Here is a brief overview to set yourself up for success:

First, find a quiet relaxing space where you feel safe to sit peacefully for thirty minutes or so. Make sure you won't be interrupted by people, pets, the phone or sudden noises—if possible. Get comfortable with the temperature of the room and have a blanket or sweater nearby in case you get cold because you will be sitting still.

Let your body settle down and your mind simmer down. Quieting your body is one thing, but quieting your mind is the part that most people have trouble achieving. Taking deep, slow breaths is one way to relax the brain; it really does change the brain waves. Don't worry too much about how you are breathing in the beginning of your attempts; the more you worry, the harder you try, and the tenser your breathing can become.

Now, add some simple movements to your breathing like bringing your shoulders up toward your ears as you inhale through the nose and then releasing the shoulders gently down as you imagine stress running down your arms, down your hands and off your fingertips while you exhale slowly with a soft sigh "haaa" through your mouth. Do this several times until your shoulders, neck and arms feel like melting butter. Take an inventory of your body and see what else is tense and make loving suggestions for it to soften and relax.

The third step is taking care of that monkey mind. Notice what kinds of thoughts continue to bug you. Your body can distract you, too. The stomach growls, which leads to wondering what's for dinner, which leads to making a grocery list, leads to... *STOP!* Gently corral your mind back to a quiet restful place of stillness (for me it's that rock resting on the bottom of the pond). You might prefer a sound or chant or the tone of a Tibetan singing bowl or even a little bell to ring to be a cue for you to re-center. Don't be surprised if you have to do it over and over.

Be gentle, but persevere. Tell your mind to *SIT* and *STAY*, just as you would do if you were training a dog! You have to understand that the mind likes to think thoughts—that's what it has always done, that's what it is good at. Be patient, and keep bringing it back to your focus word, sound, feeling or image.

The fourth step is to relax and drift into nothingness. You are in the moment, flowing along, with no more monkey mind or bothersome thoughts. You can ease into becoming part of the universe. A friend of mine likes to use perspective to get her in the mood. First, she sees herself soaring above her house, then her neighborhood, then the city, then the state, then looking down at our continent and our planet. Then from this high perspective, she imagines she is one with the galaxy. That short-circuits her thinking brain and then she finds herself floating in nothingness. Whatever works!

Don't let your practice become uncomfortable; it should be uplifting. Find out what feels best for you. Early morning meditations are best for some. 4:00 a.m. is said to be a perfect time when the world around you is still. Perhaps you can do a gratitude list before your meditation or read a poem or passage from a book that is inspiring. There are so many ideas and aids available. Let it be an adventure, as you find out what best takes you to the "peace that passeth all understanding."

Get off that hamster wheel of life; the merry-go-round of family dramas, the stresses of competition, the desires of being more, doing more, having more, the constant interplay of relationships, the exhaustion of emotions. Whew, let it all go. You need some time off! An empty mind might feel weird to you at first, but relax... and enjoy the spaciousness and lightness of being when you aren't carrying all the ego's baggage.

Even if you only get a few seconds of peace, don't disregard it, that's progress! Moments will build to minutes and one day you will find it so rewarding to mediate that it becomes an intrinsic part of your daily life. At some point you may even find yourself in a constant state of meditation. Your world will never be the same when you become a transparency for the Light.

"Keep a secret chamber of silence within yourself, where you will not let moods, trials, battles or inharmony enter...In this chamber of peace, God will visit you."

Paramahansa Yogananda

CHAPTER 23

The Wisdom of Dreams

Some people (maybe that's you), swear they don't dream, but if you have eyelids, you do. Scientists can measure how long and how frequently you dream by observing traceable REM (rapid eye movement). Your brain waves, reflected by REM, prove you are dreaming. Humans dream five to six times a night, with more dreams occurring during the early morning hours. Some people dream in technicolor and others in black and white. Some dreamers have long involved dreams, while others have snippets of images and mini-scenarios. Some people have pleasant, sometimes ecstatic dreams, while others have nightmares and many of us have both. We dream from infanthood until our last days on earth.

There is so much wisdom to be garnered from dreams; why would we ignore them?

Unfortunately, there are those who believe that dreams are just reruns of the dramas we experience during the day; a sort of recycling process helpful for a brain on overload. Others think analyzing dream information is a waste of time. What kind of help could there be in those crazy dreams—except for a good laugh? But then there are people like me, and millions more, who treasure dreams for guidance, catharsis, balance and spiritual growth. We want to understand ourselves at both the conscious and unconscious levels and our dreams help us do just that. We are the therapists who know us best and we don't charge a dime!

We can learn dream interpretation skills from various experts and discover which techniques we like best. Making dream study a priority in our lives means that we have an inner guidance system that is always there reflecting symbols and symbolic dynamics to help us understand our lives. We can also learn to integrate the dream's guidance into our waking lives by using art, writing, movement, drama, imagery, therapy and reflection to anchor its wisdom.

I have had many wonderful dreams that have given me guidance and understanding. There are some dreams that I still don't "get," but I know the message will be repeated if it is important. I love to go to sleep and know that messages will be communicated through symbols and symbolic dramas that I can look at to see what is going on with me at a deep level. It isn't always immediately clear what the dream is telling me, so I may have to let it "simmer on the back burner" for days, months or years. Thankfully, I have a great dream group I meet with every two weeks to help me interpret my dream messages. You don't have to wing it alone. Find people in your area who are interested in working with their dreams.

Many famous people paid attention to their dreams

for help in battle strategies, healings, decision making, inner guidance and problem solving. I have a friend who dreams about her next painting. There are writers who receive plots for books, inspiration for poetry, and ideas for scripts through their dreams. I've even had dreams suggest new hairstyles for me!

According to an account from a close friend of his, Abraham Lincoln had a dream that he was walking around the White House and saw a parlor room in which a dead body in a coffin was surrounded by grieving people. He asked a servant, "Who died?" and the servant answered, "The President." Too bad his dream didn't prevent him from going to the theater... but maybe that was his destiny.

Mahatma Gandhi had a dream that gave him the idea for passive resistance that helped his country overcome Britain's rule. It informed him that if he could organize the many diverse religious sects of India for a one-day peaceful protest using passive resistance, he could get Britain's attention. He relayed his idea from the dream to religious leaders who agreed to cooperate with him. This idea stopped the working class of India from going to work. With servants, transportation drivers, storekeepers and other essential workers staying home, the impact was incredible. It was a brilliant way to hold a massive, nationwide peaceful protest to show the British that India had a secret weapon all its own—passive resistance. An amazing gift of strategy from a dream.

A well-known minister, Reverend Michael Bernard Beckwith, founder of Agape International Spiritual Center, recounts a dream he had at 27 years of age which led him into the ministry and the founding of a church with over 8,000 members in California. Beckwith was headed into the field of medicine when he had his life-changing dream. It was his mountain peak spiritual experience. Now, some fifty years later, he has never looked back and still credits this dream as changing his life.

I know from my own experience that dreams have the ability to change you at a deep level. You may wake up a different person as I did one morning after having a night terror (an intense nightmare that overwhelms you with fear).

I was able to pull myself free of this night terror only by pleading to myself, *It's a dream, it's a dream, wake up*! I finally awoke, thinking my hair may have turned white because the nightmare was so terrorizing. I sobbed for a few minutes with the relief of being alive and coming back into waking reality. I went to the mirror to see who this new person was looking back at me.

I didn't know how, why or what triggered this dream, but I felt a release from a fear I had carried with me for years.

> *In the dream, I am about five years old and am in my bed in the dark. I pull my blanket, the familiar old worn one, up around my chin and wait, terrorized, for what is about to happen. Footsteps are coming down the hall. I am about to be killed. I have never felt that level of fear.*

When I woke up, a great deal of subconscious anxiety was drained from me and I felt like a wet noodle! I got ready for my day feeling like a new person even though I was weak and trembling. This dream allowed some stuck emotions to surface that needed to be expressed, and provided a release that I needed.

Running away from someone is one of the most frequent dream scenarios people have. Being naked, late for school or an appointment, falling, failing, or trying to complete a task or test, are some other popular themes that pervade our dreams. By examining our nightmares, we can learn a lot about ourselves. Once we understand the message, the nightmares will often disappear. Bringing what is unconscious to consciousness is liberating; those fears want out!

Dreams of flight can make us feel ecstatic. I miss those dreams where I would fly high over cities, trees, meadows and the ocean. As I got older, my flying dreams became rarer—much to my disappointment. It took a lot of work to get up into the air. I couldn't get much higher than the ceiling or rise only to the branches of a tree. But I found a trick that I use even today. I imagine myself jumping on a trampoline and at the high point of the jump, I concentrate on continuing to rise up into the air. Using this technique, I can still fly, but it is nothing like the dreams of my youth when I went soaring through the clouds like Superman!

Animal dreams are loaded with imagery, energy and symbolism. My dreams of animals being encased in concrete or hardened plaster came at a time when I felt paralyzed to move forward in my life. These dreams reflected how lifeless I was feeling then. By looking at these imprisoned animals, I was able to feel compassion for myself and take a look at what was making me feel stuck. I have had important dreams with lions, horses, buffalo, snakes, cats and even a platypus as symbols.

You will learn, as certain elements appear repeatedly in your dreams, that these are potent personal symbols for you. For me, a squirrel appearing in my dream means something crazy or "squirrely" is going on. The squirrel symbol is loaded with energy because of a childhood incident when a squirrel ran into our home and my mom had to get it out by chasing it with a broom. It was scary at the time because she was afraid that the squirrel could have rabies. When a squirrel shows up in my dreams, I know something "nutty" is happening in my life.

One of my favorite precognitive dreams contained an invitation to a magical worldwide event—the Harmonic Convergence. I didn't know anything about the Harmonic Convergence in 1987 until this dream came to say I was supposed to be there. Here is the dream:

I am happily getting ready for my date with an artist I've never met—a man named José Argüelles. The letters of his name are spelled out one at a time and float in the air reminding me of the smoke exhaled from the mouth of the caterpillar in Alice In Wonderland. I am at a high-quality art gallery where he has many large, beautiful abstract paintings on display. José, dressed in an impeccable white suit, arrives for our date in a white limousine. He is dark and handsome and is wearing sunglasses (at night). I realize he is blind. I am so excited—this feels so right.

When I had this dream, I had not heard of José Argüelles (an expert on Mayan culture, author and artist) and I hadn't read any reports about the Harmonic Convergence. It was only while I was talking with a friend that I learned about this world-wide New Age event being held soon.

She asked if I would be going and if I needed a ride. I interrupted her and said, "I know who the organizer is—José Argüelles—I dreamt about him the other night!"

I told my friend I had "gotten the invitation," but didn't realize it was a real happening! Now I knew I had a date with destiny—Harmonic Convergence here I come! I made sure I got to the Serpent Mound in Southern Ohio that day of August 27th, 1987 to be a part of the celebration that was timed to coordinate with astrological aspects. People were meeting at sacred sites all over the world, gathering to align their spiritual energies for peace and to open a way for communication with other beings. I wasn't sure why I had been alerted. I just knew I wasn't going to miss it for anything!

My then-husband drove at top speed for several hours over the hilly country roads from Dayton, Ohio to the Serpent Mound. He was excited for me when I told him about my dream and I think he expected I might be abducted. (Maybe he was hoping!) Thankfully, we made the trip in one piece and entered the festivities through a rainbow balloon gateway. It was a hippie gathering with dancing, chanting, meditating and peaceful loving vibes. Helicopters buzzed overhead and the local sheriff, flanked by his deputies, stomped around to intimidate us, but nothing could ruin the magic of the day.

My 8 year old daughter and I sat in the grass near the mound and drew meditative mandalas to celebrate the day. We joined hands with others to form a circle at dusk to anchor our prayers for peace. It was awesome being a part of something so special at that unique place (Serpent Mound is one of the few serpent-shaped effigies in the world). I was grateful that my dream made sure I was invited to the celebration. You can read more about the Harmonic Convergence in the book: *Ancient Voices, Current Affairs*, by Steven McFadden.

I enjoy a New Year's Day ritual of going over my dreams of the past year, looking for any patterns, emotional themes, recurring symbols or premonitions that I might have missed at the time of the dream. Reading these recorded dreams again and remembering the waking life experiences that I had during the year helps me see the whole picture of that time. This is an interesting way to follow up on any guidance I may have missed at the time of the dream.

I have worked with my dreams in a variety of ways through the years. Whatever technique I choose, whether working alone or with others, dream decoding begins with one thing: writing down the dream. Sometimes I use pens that have different colors in them accessed by a simple click at the top of the pen. I might circle the action words in one color and the emotions in another, underline recurring symbols in another color and take day notes in another. Day notes are about whatever is going on in waking life at the time. There is often a correlation between the dream and real time events.

I keep my dream notebook and pen on my bedside

table and record my dreams first thing in the morning. This is the best time for me to write everything down while it is still fresh and clear. On a busy day, I will jot down a few key words so I will remember the dream and work on it later. If I don't do this, I quite often forget and then worry that I lost an important message.

Upon awakening, a good practice would be to take note of how you feel and what position your body is in. Lie still for a moment and recall the dream if you have the time. Even if you don't remember all parts of the dream, write down what you can. Sometimes later in the day the whole dream will come back to you. If you only remember a fragment, take note of it. As we often say in my dream group: every "snippet" is packed with information.

Basic dream tools are your notebook, pen and a light to use in the dark (a little book light or small flashlight) or a recording device. At times, I have been so sleepy that all I could get down were a few scribbles of words, hoping they would be enough to remind me of the dream in the morning. Some people prefer to speak their dream into their phones or a tape recorder and transcribe them later. Find out what works best for you.

Once you have the dream recorded, you can separate out all the elements and look at each piece of the puzzle individually. Objects, people, animals, colors, dynamics, actions, emotions, puns, humorous situations, your favorite pet phrases, slang, songs, cultural references, or family jokes are all rich material the dream-spirit uses to communicate with us.

Think of yourself as a detective following the clues

and solving the mystery of who you are and what your subconscious is working on. Dreams are often reflecting a problem or situation that is coming up or being triggered in the present. It could be a recent drama or one that goes all the way back to childhood.

It is very important to record your feelings in the dream. Basic emotions are happy, sad, afraid and angry. But there are many variations like: confusion, shame, arrogance, shyness, detachment, frustration, agitation, grief, deceit, desire, rage—and many more. Let yourself "feel" your way back into the dream and see what the emotions reveal.

Some interesting questions to ask yourself are: What is the dream asking of you? To complete something? Solve or challenge something? Look at some situation or person in a different way? Does the dream relate to anything that is happening in your life now or in the past? How would you like to change the dream? Perhaps by confronting that monster who is chasing you, you can find out who it is and why it is chasing you. If you continue to have that dream, try talking to the monster or even *becoming* the monster to understand the message of why it appeared in your dream.

Look for the general mood of the dream along with what parts have the highest and lowest emotional energy. The lighting (dark, bright, gray) and atmosphere (sunny, gray, cloudy, cold, rainy) of the dream are always things that stand out for me, along with the colors in the setting and in the clothes people are wearing. I am very tuned in to color symbology. Lately, I have had a lot of brown-toned dreams which I interpret as a muddy dark atmosphere. They have unpleasant themes every time because for me, brown is a very undesirable color that I find quite depressing.

You can look up the meaning of symbols in a dream or symbol book, but more importantly, ask yourself what that symbol means to you. If you dream of a dog, do you love dogs or fear them? What kind of dog is it? How does the dog act? Is it acting out of character? Is it conveying an emotion? A dream or symbol book might say dreaming of a dog is about devotion and loyalty, but if you were once bitten by a dog, your feelings may be charged with mistrust. Remember, it always goes back to your experience and what feels right to you. Be alert for an "aha" reaction—when you *know that you know* without question what it means.

Another example of the many meanings within a symbol is the ocean or water appearing in your dream. If there are big waves it could mean a fearful, turbulent time or event. If you like to swim in the ocean, you may find the ocean to be a positive, playful symbol. If you don't like to swim in the ocean and find yourself there, your dream may be saying you're in "deep water" or "out of your depth"! You could be "drowning" in feelings, or if you are happily floating along you could be "going with the flow." A raging river has a different message for you than a mud puddle or a clear pond. Water is a wonderful symbol to work with, but if it is flowing over a dam it may mean you have to urinate!

When you have a symbol that repeats itself over and over again, take note! You can add it to your dream glossary of symbols in your dream notebook.

This glossary can become part of your personal dream vocabulary. Your dreaming mind has found you are paying attention to symbols that it likes to use, which is good news for you. Make a list of these and you will find your subconscious will use these symbols even more now that it sees you are listening to them.

I often dream of swimming pools which are a spiritual, happy and fun symbol for me. The day is sunny, the pool is clean and sparkling and I can't wait to get in it. I am happy and expectant of that glorious swim I am about to take. Another recurring dream is that I am lost in a huge hotel complex with many floors, stairways, elevators and halls and I don't have my room key, nor do I remember my room number. I lose my bearings and wander around in the maze feeling angry and stupid. These dreams are a reflection of confusion and remind me that I need to ask someone for help—a major theme in my dreams.

When you join a dream group or have a partnership with another dream worker, you don't have to wing it. There are many books that explain a variety of techniques and formats you can use. *Dream Work*, by Jeremy Taylor, is one of my favorite books and there are many authors such as Patricia Garfield, Gayle Delaney, Robert Hoss, Tallulah Lyons, Robert Johnson and Justina Lasley who can guide and inspire you.

Taking turns, with one person sharing per meeting, is what most groups do, making sure that everyone has a chance to share week by week. If someone has a nightmare or a dream that begs to be addressed immediately, you can negotiate the time and see what the group consensus is to let that person speak. Or an appointment could be made with another dream group member for a session outside of the group.

The opening few minutes of the meeting may involve a welcome and a few minutes of relaxation and centering. A word about the intention of the group and reminder that "what is said here, stays here" could be next. Have the dreamer tell the dream in first person and in the present tense, as well as the title of the dream and the date it appeared. Let the dreamer tell the dream all the way through before asking any questions. She can read it from her notebook or speak it from memory.

Clarification comes next. The participants in the group then ask questions to get clarity on the dream. This will help the dreamer, too, in remembering more details. Questions from the group might include: what are the feelings or emotions in the dream, what are the high energy points of the dream, what kind of dog (for example) is it, what is it doing, why isn't the owner paying attention to it, and how did it get on the diving board? Then you may want to ask the dreamer to become the dog and let it speak. To do this, ask one person to take the position of relaxing the dreamer and leading her back into the dream. This is done gently by asking the dreamer to close her eyes, sense the dog and then become the dog.

The group will wait until the dreamer says he or she feels like the dog and is ready to speak as the dog. Questions are then asked, like what kind of dog are you, what is your function or job, what do you like or not like about yourself, why are you on a diving board, how do you feel about it, etc... At the end, ask if the dog has anything else to say or a message for the dreamer. Thank the dog and the dreamer, and slowly ask the dreamer to return to his or her body. Someone who has been recording this segment can then read it back to the dreamer. Perhaps the dog really does not like the position it is in, being obedient and having to perform something way out of its comfort zone. Then we wait for the dreamer to make his or her own conclusions about what has been gleaned from the dream.

Respect is always given to the dreamer's interpretation of the dream, for he or she is the author, actors, casting agent and audience for the dream. Others can help you unwrap the dream, but no one has the right to take the gift away from you by insisting they know what it means. They are able to give suggestions, talk about the symbols, refer to what it would mean for them and ask the dreamer questions, but no one is to say, "I know the correct, only and perfect interpretation of this dream."

At the end of the meeting, each member can express what the dream meant to them by saying, "If this were my dream, I would interpret it as…" Other people's dreams have messages for everyone in the group.

Another powerful way to work with dreams is to perform a reenactment with the support of your trusted dream circle. For several years, I experienced repeated dreams of shame that found me in a very uncomfortable situation:

I am in an office or an aisle of K-Mart, some public place, going to the toilet in front of everyone! I am so embarrassed to find myself in such an awkward position. I fluff out my full skirt to hide the toilet and

*try to act like nothing unusual is happening. I know I
am not fooling anybody and I am filled with shame.*

At a meeting of a dream group of women I knew well,
I asked if I might act out this dream in front of them. I
got a chair and put it in the middle of the group and sat
down pretending it was a toilet. I let my mind go back
into that awful situation. At first, I laughed nervously,
then I felt weird, then relieved when I saw no one was
shocked or shaming me. This led to a neutral feeling and
a release of laughter. What a relief about relieving myself!
Now I rarely have that dream, so I know that some of my
shame issues are being resolved.

You will have dreams that show you your dark side;
something ugly or embarrassing you don't want to look
at consciously. *That's me? I have those feelings inside me?*
You might see yourself robbing or hurting someone. I
had a dream about a girlfriend of mine who was having
a happy romance. In my dream, I went to her home and
cut off her pretty long hair! There was a part of me that
didn't want to acknowledge my jealousy.

I once had a dream where I was violently strangling
my father and bashing his head against hard ceramic
tiles. That was an intense dream, but I am thankful for
it because it discharged some of the negative feelings I
had for him. My relationship with my father continues
in my dreams even though he has been dead for years.

I had this dream recently:

*I am sitting on my dad's lap with my head on his
shoulder. I feel protected and loved. I am comfortable*

and he is, too. We are soaking up what we never had between us.

Another recent dream had me walking up to him and giving him a long hug. Something is being healed between us. Some people report dreams in which their relationships with others have a life of their own continuing on for years and evolving toward healing. I am sure this is happening with me and my father and I hope that someday it will happen with my mother and me, too.

Recurring dreams are trying to get your attention! An example of a very repetitive dream of mine is on the theme of trying to get home:

I am somewhere with people, maybe an outdoor bar. I want to go home and realize I have no car. It is too far to walk, I don't have the money to call a cab, I don't have a cell phone to call someone to come and get me and there is no one to ask for a ride! I am left feeling helpless.

I studied these dreams for years, always thinking they had something to do with trying to go home (safety) or to another state of mind. Home is a loaded symbol because it is so important to everyone. I thought this dream represented my trying to return to that place of safety and familiarity, but this dream kept coming until I asked myself, *where are my resources in this dream?* I don't have anything to take care of myself: no money, no car, no purse, no phone, no friends with me to help. In a few dreams I had a bicycle, but home was too far to go on a bike. I could walk, but it was through a neighborhood that was too dark and dangerous. I began to see that I was a victim of my situation.

Suddenly it occurred to me: *why didn't I have what I needed to take care of myself? Is this how I function in my waking life? Am I prepared to take care of myself in an emergency? Is there a child-part of me feeling helpless instead of feeling like a competent adult?*

I decided to try something different the next time I had this dream. I vowed to have a resource with me. It took a few tries, but finally when I found myself back in the dream and it was time to go home, I didn't panic. I still didn't have a car or a phone on me, but I asked a fellow at the bar sitting next to me if I could use his phone to call for a ride home. He gladly loaned me his phone and I called somebody for help. Another time I found I had my phone with me and called a cab, but had no money to pay for the taxi. Then I realized that I could take care of the payment once I got home. In my dream, I was figuring out how to deal with the situation and not be a victim of it.

Looking at my waking life, I realized how often I left home without being completely prepared. Yes, I locked the door and had my car keys, but I needed to look at other resources. The youth today call it "adulting." I started taking the time before I left the house to check if I had my phone and it was charged. I made sure I had the directions, the money I needed and had given myself sufficient time. Once I began doing this, my nighttime dreams of being stuck somewhere disappeared. I love how these two parts of my conscious and unconscious life worked out the problem.

Another example of a recurring dream that enabled me to take action in my daily life and effect change in the course of the dreams is of my being pinned down by a heavy man. I felt his weight on me as I struggled and screamed. After years of these overwhelming dreams, I began to take a stand in the dream. First, I locked the bedroom door and threatened to call the police on him. It took a few years of working with this dream until eventually I stood up against his abuse. It happened little by little until finally he didn't dare try to overpower me. I was empowered and he knew it. The evolution of these dreams was the result of years of therapy and finding my voice.

A friend of mine was disturbed at his recurring dreams about taking his dad to the airport. He was a little boy in the dream. All I had to do was ask him about his childhood to find out that he had in fact gone with his mother to take his father to the airport many times for military duty. Once he talked about this with me and acknowledged his sadness as a child, the dreams stopped. Our emotions will pervade our dreams when they need to be examined. Just acknowledging an incident can release the pattern or trauma stuck in our psyche. Our dreams are always moving us toward wholeness.

My sexual abuse dreams began when I was forty. My therapists were always asking me to explore the subject, but I refused to go there. I denied it could have anything to do with me. Here is the very first dream that gently opened the door on the subject:

My uncle presents me with an article about sexual abuse printed in a newspaper. I take the paper and read the article. I have no reaction to the dream since the story isn't about me or anyone I know. I read the information in a detached way and feel no connection.

The brain, I have learned, will be careful not to give you too much, too soon. It's a precautionary measure that your mind takes to make sure you are ready to handle the secrets it holds. Opening Pandora's box can also be triggered by events or by the age of the children you have as it correlates to the age you were when the abuse happened to you. Sometimes the timing can be the result of working with a therapist who provides you with a safe place and person to tell.

You can have premonitions in your dreams. A friend of mine had a dream where she was standing in her front yard with her little grandson and a car coming down her street jumped the curb where he was standing and hit him. The next day, when she found herself in a real-life situation repeating the dream scenario, she knew what to do. She grabbed the little boy and threw him out of the way at the very moment a car traveled over the curb and drove into her yard. It was just as her dream had foretold.

You can have compensatory dreams that the psyche gives you to keep you in balance. I may not admit to myself that I want a boyfriend, but my dreaming self may produce one. I had a great new love recently, the eminent scholar and author, Joseph Campbell! I might dream I have beautiful clothes when my wardrobe is lacking, a banquet served to me when I am on a diet, or I will take a trip when I am feeling stuck at home—all dreams that are filling a void.

When I was considering divorce, I had many dreams of being on one boat and seeing my then-husband on another—and we were traveling in opposite directions. I felt great sadness as the dreams continued and the boats kept getting farther and farther away from each other. I was preparing through my dreams for our separation.

For ten years after my divorce, I had dreams that I was with my ex-husband and we were looking for a new home. It was my psyche's attempt to give us another chance. We were so happy to find our new place and fix up the house and then... we remembered. He was married to someone else now! The new wife was never going to go along with this! Then, as the dream continued, we tried to figure out how to handle the "fly in the ointment." I didn't consciously want to get back in a relationship with him, but evidently my psyche had different ideas! You may be surprised at how other parts of you are experiencing a transition.

Recently, I had another dream of my ex-husband that was sweet and comforting:

It is night and we are standing outside together looking up at stars sparkling across a dark midnight blue sky. We are admiring a huge pink satin bow floating among the stars. It is quite amazing and beautiful.

My interpretation is that we were looking at our marriage and the gift it gave us—two wonderful daughters and many good years; years that were tied up with a big beautiful pink bow.

Whatever you decipher from your dreams can be added to your knowledge of yourself: your motives, desires, dynamics, fears, along with what needs to be worked up and out of your psyche. Your dreams are mirroring deep issues that may be keeping you from living your best and most authentic life.

There are all kinds of dream groups if you don't want to work alone. Some are casual while others take on a more formal approach. I suggest a group with no more than 8 participants. I appreciate a well-run meeting where people show up on time and don't talk over each other. I particularly like the *Haden Institute's* approach that regards dreams and dream work as sacred.

You will have to discover what works best for you. All dream groups have as a first commandment, "What is said here, stays here." A second commandment is to never take the dream away from the person having it. Dream group etiquette is not to talk over anyone, do not monopolize the group, be focused, respectful, and do not have side conversations or try to "fix" anyone.

Sometimes it is difficult not to blurt out exactly what you believe the dream means (as *you* interpret it). You have to stop yourself! One of the most important parts of the process is letting the dreamer "unwrap" the gift of their dreams.

It may take some time for you to feel comfortable in the group. Don't make any hasty judgements in deciding whether to stay or go. You may be like me, wanting to feel safe before I open up and get comfortable sharing my dreams with the group. A good dream group will honor the dream process and the leader will respect everyone there. Continued and faithful attendance helps the group to "gel."

Dreams are also a way to become aware of what your physical issues are in life. How does this tie in with cancer? Symbols of health issues often appear in your dreams to warn you of future problems. Dream work is another tool to help you figure out what is going on beneath the surface of your consciousness. Through dreams, you will see your anger, sadness, hopes and fears regarding a life-threatening situation played out. Symbols and scenarios through dreams can reflect information to help you understand the illness, identify what emotions it brings up for you and what to do with those feelings. You may see solutions or find solace. Dreams shed a light on what needs to be acknowledged and examined.

The parasite dream I had before I found the swollen lymph node disgusted me to the point where I avoided working on it. Other than that dream and a few dreams reflecting my fear of death, my cancer was fairly silent. I wondered why I didn't get some kind of definitive dream about the cancer to give me a warning of what was to come. It wasn't until 2 years after my diagnosis (in 2021) that I found the following dream in a sheaf of papers that I was going through while packing to move. It was among several recorded dreams I had torn out of my dream diaries to alert myself to work on later. Here is the dream:

(August 3, 2015) *I am in a hospital setting with another woman who is younger than me. We are both being examined. We are on exam tables naked. She is going to have a baby and is moved to another spot. I am very upset. I feel shame, vulnerability and anger. I am told I have cancer. I don't like all the people who are crowded in this small room. I feel claustrophobic.*

This scene was played out in real life in 2019 when I found myself in the tiny exam room at Hollings Cancer Center. I often had three people in the room with me while I was being examined.

What advice could I have taken from this dream? Perhaps, I could have begun having Pap smears done since I had stopped at age 65. I don't know if it would have changed anything. The experience of cancer seems to have been my destiny.

Recently, I interviewed Tallulah Lyons, dream worker and author, who has worked with many cancer patients through the Cancer Project sponsored by the International Association of Dreams.

The Cancer Project's dream circles, led by Tallulah Lyons and Wendy Pannier, were held in hospital settings with the intention of helping patients deal with the stress, pain and uncertainty of disease and possible death from cancer.

As a result of the success of these dream circles, Tallulah wrote the book, *Dreams and Guided Imagery: Gifts for Transforming Illness and Crisis*. The techniques covered in her book include: dialoguing with the dream, working with symbols, re-entry and re-scripting the dream, how caregivers can give feedback to the dreamer, how to use guided imagery while working with symbols from the dream, guided dream imagery scripts, how to run a dream group (format and ethics), a great appendix and the unique opportunity to experience a dream circle as it operates. Her writing style makes the dream group come alive for the reader.

Tallulah explained that she fell in love with dreams as a five-year-old and her interest has never waned. "As a child, I was always in touch with my dreams. My childhood was rocky and I had to cope and build a protective world around myself. I always felt very connected to something much bigger than myself," she explains.

Lyons reported that her interest in dreams and all things spiritual were threads that wound their way throughout her life as she pursued careers as an English Literature Teacher, Special Education Consultant, Tutor, and Haden Institute certified Dream Facilitator.

In 2003, the Cancer Project was offered to hospitals as an integrative therapy for patients. Tallulah and Wendy discovered that their dream circle sessions decreased feelings of anxiety and gave participants a feeling of control over their lives along with a desire to live fully in spite of cancer.

"I treasure my years of doing dream work with cancer patients," Lyons recalled. "Everyone's dream brought gifts for the whole group. I've witnessed people who, though they may be dying, are able to get in touch with their undying spirit."

Lyons experienced a mid-life crisis in the mid 1990's that she describes as a loss of faith. "I was dropping into a dark place of depression. My dreams were full of blood and gore. They were so vivid, showing me what a bad place I was in. My dreams told me to shape up or die!" As this "dark night of the soul" was threatening to overtake her, Tallulah chose to go into Jungian Analysis for ten years where she received help unraveling her descent.

"I finally found out who I really was when I started to do dream work with cancer patients," Tallulah recounted. She brought to it all her talents as an artist, educator, wife, mother and seasoned dream worker. "By following the path of dreams," she said, "I was on the road to become the person I was meant to be."

Dreams can release stress, help us deal with limitations, and open us up to healing and a sense of connection and meaning, Tallulah explains in her book. Sharing dreams relieves some of the emotional stress and brings support for those dealing with cancer and other life-threatening diseases. According to Tallulah, "Dream work addresses death, crisis, and trauma—allowing people to live fully no matter the circumstances."

Tallulah designed her own method for dreamers to work with their images and symbols through guided imagery. "Guided imagery is a natural process that helps us further explore the dreams' symbols and messages. I weave the two together (nighttime dreams and waking guided symbol exploration) creating a bridge to waking life."

Lyons believes that the imagery of symbols is the language of the deep self that moves us closer to the core of our being. Cancer can also force a deep examination of ourselves, therefore dream and symbol work are a natural complement.

"I am so lucky to have found dreamwork so early. My dreams have shaped my whole life." Tallulah, retired from her dream circles at hospitals and now 82, is still involved with three dream groups that she attends online.

Dreams and Guided Imagery contains several guided imagery scripts to follow—even one to help the dreamer transform a nightmare. Lyons recommends 30 minutes of uninterrupted time for meditative dreaming. This is a hypnagogic experience that invites imagery to come to the surface of the mind. Healing images can be used in daily meditations and to bring the dreamer a sense of peace and connection. Art, movement and writing exercises can be integrated to create a connection between dreams and spiritual healing.

Thank you, Tallulah, for the interview and for writing your wonderful book, *Dreams and Guided Imagery: Gifts for Transforming Illness and Crisis*. What you have provided for cancer patients both in person and through your book is a way to heal. From your childhood years until the present, your sharing of dreams, symbols and imagery has given seekers many tools to understand their cancer journey.

CHAPTER 24

Intuition and Guidance

Intuition—is it an animal instinct? Coming from our subconscious mind? Communication from our souls? We call it a hunch, a nudge, a sixth sense, a premonition, the shivers, goosebumps, gut feelings, a feeling in our heart or an impulse coming from "somewhere out there." Intuition can be all these things and more.

I've read that Oprah Winfrey lives her life by using her intuition, saying, "Intuition is the voice of God. It doesn't lie." She describes her intuitive feelings welling up inside her as a vibratory force felt in every cell of her body.

Actor, author and deep thinker, Alan Alda, describes intuition very poetically saying, "At times you have to leave the city of your comfort and go into the wilderness of your intuition. What you will discover will be wonderful. What you will discover is yourself."

I believe we all have intuition, which is a sixth sense that can be added to the five we already have. Intuition can help you live a better life; it's an internal guidance system. Decisions regarding health, career, business, parenting, survival and relationships are all better decisions when intuition is added to the process.

Let me give you a few examples of what intuition *is* and is *not.*

Recently, I realized that some of what I thought of as intuition was actually coming from my rational brain. I have a very vigilant brain which developed from my childhood strategy of trying to keep myself safe in a crazy family atmosphere that often felt dangerous. In order to stay safe, I had to be able to connect the dots of what was happening or about to happen and what I should do, so quickly that it didn't feel like thinking at all. I thought of it as intuition. I have since realized that I take the details of what is going on around me, add them up at lightning speed and make a decision based on the facts—that is a left-brain skill and protective mechanism.

I can go into a gathering or situation and immediately sense the mood, pick up on signs of discontent, trouble, uncertainty and decide within seconds if I am safe or not. This is not true intuition, since I am guided by observations of minute facial expressions, body postures, voice inflections, conversations and other clues all pertaining to whether or not I am safe. This is assessed by my brain in milli-seconds and although it seems like intuition is guiding me, it is not.

Like a detective, who is trained to discern signs of possible guilt from the smallest twitch of a suspect's eye, speech inflections, skin reactions, and an imperceptible shrug of the shoulders, I pick up on those signs in order to make my decision of whether it is time to leave the party or safe to stay.

We all have intuition, but for some it is a dormant gift just waiting to be awakened. We may have to coax it into our lives and exercise it to make it strong. When it appears, recognize and acknowledge it. It will begin to feel quite natural and as something to be trusted.

Intuition has been known to save lives, keep us out of a disastrous business situation or a doomed relationship. How many times have we heard people say, "Oh I knew that guy was trouble," or "I had a feeling I shouldn't sign that contract," or "I never trusted her—I don't know why…" A warning might be a subtle shiver that runs down your spine or a heavy sense of dread that says, "This isn't right! Something's off! She's lying!"

When you get that feeling, do not get into that car, swim in that river, take that path, trust that person, go to that party—the list goes on and on. Pay attention to that voice or nudge wherever it comes from. It may not be logical, it may not be the most comfortable choice, but take it seriously—it could save your life.

I was once scammed on the phone by a caller who was pretending to be my husband. He was so friendly and casual that I was actually fooled. My intuition suddenly sent a feeling of alarm that went through me like a surge of electricity. I threw the phone across the room. I didn't logically figure out I was being scammed, but my inner alert system knew exactly what to do.

Recently, a friend told me of the scary situation she had years ago with her baby boy who was projectile vomiting. After examining the infant, her doctor said it wasn't anything to worry about and sent her and the baby home. Once there, she took a moment to listen to her inner maternal intuition and she "knew" his advice wasn't right. She got back into the car and headed to the hospital where an emergency doctor immediately diagnosed and treated the infant for a dangerous life-threatening condition. I like the end of this story; a few days later she went back to the first doctor's office to let him know what had happened. On her way out, she advised the people in the waiting room, "If I had followed this doctor's advice, I would have lost my son!"

Parents are known for sensing if something isn't right with their children. Part of that wisdom comes from being around the child 24/7, but intuition is at work, too. Parents are fine-tuned to their families and will get a "hunch" that something's wrong even when their children are forty or fifty years old! No matter what the age, go ahead and make that phone call and ask, "Are you okay, Honey?"

When my daughter was in Germany, I suddenly got the urge to call her. "Anything interesting happening in your life today," I asked, wondering about the strange wording I was using. "Mom! I just took a pregnancy test and it was positive!" she exclaimed. I was the first to know.

Our need to protect our kids is always there. A few months ago, I noticed a shrub in Shanen's yard that was overgrown and needed tending. I just "knew" something dangerous was living in there and told her to be extra careful when she cleaned up that bushy area. "I'm sensing a snake," I warned. Tidying up her yard soon after, she began to carefully hack away at the weeds around that corner bush and a stream of angry yellow jackets spewed out from their underground nest. She was on alert and was able to back away quickly. A few nights later, we saw a snake slither into that same bush. You might say it was a logical assumption—her yard is the perfect place for critters, but every time I looked at that bush, I got an "off" feeling and an image of a snake came to me. I do not censor myself when something comes to mind, I say it and take the risk of sounding crazy! Luckily, she took my warning seriously and was prepared to retreat when she stirred up those wasps.

Intuition can put you on alert when you are in danger. This happened to me many years ago, but I recall the incident like it was yesterday. When Shanen was about five or six years of age, I took her to a large wooded nature park for an afternoon walk. When we got to the parking lot and exited our car, I noticed a guy pulling up in his car at the far end of the lot. We were the only cars there which gave me a funny feeling realizing the park was empty on this mid-week day. We didn't get very far on the path down to the creek when I felt uncomfortable, restless, and felt eyes on me giving me goosebumps. I tried to brush off the feeling since my daughter and I were both looking forward to our nature hike. However, I kept sensing something wasn't safe and my intuition told me to leave.

With the hair on the back of my neck bristling, I grabbed my little girl's arm and told her to walk fast. "We're leaving now!" My intuition was screaming—*go, go, go, go!* We got into my car and I spun out in the gravel as I made my getaway. When I look back on that incident, I still get a funny feeling. I am thankful I trusted my intuition. If it is a warning, it will usually persist and even if it is illogical, I would advise you to act on the side of safety like I did. Better safe than sorry.

Intuition, or a metaphysical event, can come in words like it did for my mother. Mom didn't tell this story for 25 years because she said it was so special to her. It happened decades ago in New York City when she heard a voice as she was unlocking her apartment door. Out of the blue, a deep thundering voice said, "Be still and know that I AM GOD!" She looked around shocked. No neighbors were in sight! It shook her to her core. Without a doubt, she knew God had spoken to her. She told me that her investment in the dramas of her human relationships was never as intense again. Knowing God was in charge was the reminder she needed at that time.

I also have heard a voice coming from outside myself. In February 2020, I awoke to a clear voice saying: "Prepare for change!" I told my daughter that could mean anything, since life was all about change. I even laughed it off. Little did I know, there was a big change coming up—Covid-19!

Another time, I was fretting and frustrated over the slow healing of my knee replacement and a voice came to me saying, "Healing is NOT progressive!" What did that mean? I thought about it and realized I expected healing to be linear, in stages, as the physical therapist had explained to me. This new message was reassuring, telling me that my healing would not follow a step-by-step progression—and it didn't.

People express delight as they get the "shivers," when the hairs on their arms raise up alerting them to pay extra attention to whatever is happening at the moment. "Gee," they'll say, as they rub their forearms, "I just got angel bumps!" Currently, it seems like everyone is getting this reaction; I've even seen Oprah Winfrey on television acknowledging her "angel bumps."

What seems to be intuition could be feelings that come from a place of trauma. I was afraid to fly for many years and believed it was my intuition telling me my plane was going to crash. I was so terrified of this fiery death that I felt fear deep into every fiber of my being every time I had to go on an airplane trip. Finally, it got so bad, I decided airplanes were not for me—even after having numerous safe plane trips.

It wasn't my intuition or a premonition, I realized later, but the experience of a childhood trip on an airplane with my mother that prompted such extreme fear. As we flew into New York City, there was a severe storm with lightning crashing all around us. Our plane circled around and around a bay near the airport, unable to land for several hours. That trauma, experienced at ten years old, was embedded in me and triggered every time I flew. For many years, I wrote an updated will before I took off on an airplane trip and bought some high-quality chocolate bars to take with me on the plane. If I was going to die, I wanted to have chocolate in my mouth on the way down!

My decision to stop flying worked for a while, but it wasn't practical. I thought about getting hypnotized or taking one of those desensitization workshops airlines used to give to fearful flyers. I knew that I was much more likely to die in a car trip than from a plane crash, but knowing that fact did not help. Then, came the real test. I desperately wanted to travel from the West Coast to the East Coast and a plane trip would get me there in an afternoon, but terror welled up in me once again and I decided I couldn't fly. I just couldn't do it! Instead, I took a bus. Traveling for five days and nights across the continent from California to Virginia Beach cured me of my fear—I called it "Greyhound Bus Aversion Therapy"!

I decided that death from a plane crash was better than that experience! It took me several days after I disembarked from the bus until my body stopped moving. The experiences I had on that trip (including meeting the original Aunt Jemima as a seat-mate) could fill a book. Even though I still get nervous about flying, I no longer torment myself over it. I realize that what I thought of as a premonition of death was a re-lived trauma from my scary childhood flight. However, I still buy good chocolate to have with me, just in case.

Don't be tricked into believing something is intuition when it is a trauma being triggered or perhaps something you want to do anyway: "I knew in my heart he (or she) was the one for me." How many of us have said that! We are being swept away by that old trickster called romance. Then, the night before the wedding, reality sets in. Cold feet (backing away) before marriage is a common occurrence, but it doesn't always mean it's your intuition telling you it's doomed. I'm just saying... divorce rates are outrageously high. Decreased temperature in your feet might literally be the intuitive sign your body is giving you to get out while you can!

I was uncertain before I married my first husband,

but felt it was my destiny to marry him (maybe it was). My common sense told me he wasn't a good choice, but I was young and blamed it on hormones. I should have listened to my mother, who said she felt like crying out, "Save yourself!" during the entire wedding service. What can I say, Mom…I JUST HAD TO DO IT! (And she was right, divorce followed in two years).

Women's intuition is sometimes regarded as a feminine wile. I believe women are more aware of their hunches because they are biologically attuned to subtle changes in their bodies. Women have to pay attention to their physicality (menstruation, pregnancy) in ways men do not. Perhaps men have as many insights as women, but are not permitted in our culture to acknowledge them because hunches are not logical and may seem "silly," not coming from a recognized or authoritative source. I enjoy this quote from Farrah Fawcett: "God gave women intuition and femininity. Used properly, the combination easily jumbles the brain of any man I've ever met." I know, as an intuitive woman, I jumbled the brain of my scientist ex-husband too many times to count.

I have experienced guidance coming from dreams, symbols, insights, revelations, meditation, synchronicity, looking at what and whom I am attracting, noting the songs that keep repeating in my head, and a word or name that pops up over and over. However, I do caution anyone who can't live without a sign to act on may be taking it too far. If you are hearing a voice that goes on and on, becomes angry at you, accuses, blames and gives messages that are hurtful to you, then you are not experiencing intuition but something unhealthy. If inner voices are tormenting or confusing you, this may be a form of mental illness that needs to be checked out with a therapist or your doctor.

Going deep into your soul through reflection, meditation, dream study or just being mindful of how life is sending you guidance are all ways to strengthen that connection with intuition. Pay attention to your body's clues and cues. You may discover you get a cold chill when you think of someone or your heart may feel light or heavy when you enter someone's home. You may feel enlivening or deadening energy by a decision you make or a person around you. You may start to repeat some gossip and feel like you get a tap on the head, your mind goes blank, or you begin to cough or choke. That tells me to shut up!

Listen and learn how to connect these feelings to your life. I realized a long time ago that when I hit my head on an opened kitchen cupboard door, it wasn't an accident. At that very moment, I needed to stop and examine my thoughts. My inner sensor/censor was telling me, *Okay, it's time for you to stop thinking those negative thoughts!*

As I have matured, I have become more in touch with different aspects of myself. Listening to the guidance coming from all around me is a way of life now. And I keep that connection vital by journaling, studying my dreams, writing down my feelings, discussing revelations or quandaries with some treasured friends and I might do some art therapy for insights.

By looking at the symbols given to me each day, the feelings that are coming up, and the synchronicities that happen (sometimes called "Godwinks"), I can consider how unseen forces operate in my life. Occasionally, when journaling, I will write with my non-dominant hand which is a technique I learned from *The Power of the Other Hand*, an excellent book by Lucia Capacchione. This form of writing accesses my right brain where emotions, spiritual direction and my inner child reside. All these practices, including meditation, help me become more aware of how to trust that my life is unfolding as it should.

However, just because I receive inner guidance doesn't mean my life is always smooth sailing. Recently, I made a decision I felt was divinely guided. It came from an impulse that I was sure was for my highest good. I needed a roommate and had a friend who needed to find a place to live. We discussed it and a reassuring symbol occurred while we were on the phone—two hawks flew directly over my head, then turned and playfully circled around me at close range. I judged it as a confirmation! I was happy—until the situation I thought would work out perfectly backfired. (COVID came into our lives and we weren't on the same page regarding how to handle it.) *How could this have happened*, I wondered, *wasn't my intuition guiding me to my highest good?*

Therein lies the tricky part. We all want the pleasant path in life and we assume soul guidance will always lead us there. I wanted a cozy living situation, but instead I got an opportunity to practice standing up for myself! It is hard to accept that our highest good (meaning soul growth) can sometimes be downright painful. If something doesn't work out to our perceived advantage, we often judge it as negative. Growth can be hard work. In this instance, I accepted that the situation worked out perfectly. Oh, how we love those opportunities for growth!

As you pay attention to your life, you will find out how intuition manifests for you. It could be an inner impulse, or a whisper in your ear; you do not have to know its origin. It could be an animal messenger. It could be a person you keep running into, a word that pops up in your reading or a thought that keeps telling you something.

A few days after my mother died, a close friend of hers called me and said, "You are not going to believe this! I am sitting in my car in a busy parking lot waiting to go in to an appointment and there is a peacock strutting around in front of my bumper! I believe it's your mother saying, 'Hi!'" I chuckled and agreed. My mother would pick a peacock, a favorite bird symbol for her. She had the peacock motif in her apartment including a peacock feather fan on her wall. She also enjoyed wearing fabulous peacock feather earrings and showing off her beauty for all to admire. I think Mom was there in symbolic form strutting her stuff.

My personal experience is that I do not get a heart flutter, tingle, shiver or bumps as many do, but my intuition usually manifests as a voice, insistent and to the point, or as a mental interruption to whatever I am thinking at the time, or those head whacks from the kitchen cupboards. I also pay attention to the words that come to me out of the blue on license plates, billboards or in one instance on the back of a truck I was following.

There it was, my message for the day. I read these printed words painted in purple on the back of a dump truck: "Don't Let Your Problems Pollute the World." I was taken back. I had never thought that my problems could do that. Well, somebody had this realization and was motivated enough to take a paint brush and write that message to be transported along the highways. It gave me pause to think about the negativity we dump into the collective consciousness. Wisdom is everywhere and how appropriate it was to see it written on a *dump* truck!

Recently, I predicted (only to myself) three deaths a few days before they happened. Two were acquaintances and one was a celebrity. This is new for me and I am not sure I like it. Every time I think of someone several times, I begin to wonder if their death is imminent. I got that feeling about my aunt recently and made sure I called her.

Sometimes, intuition or guidance comes through in dreams. I write down my dreams almost daily and have for decades. I think about them throughout the day, mulling over what message, insight or guidance is in them waiting for me to figure out. That magical moment between sleep and waking, called hypnagogia, is a time when the veil between conscious and subconscious is very thin. Being aware of this time can help attune oneself to a higher vibration. Along with meditation, these are times to "dial" into a clearer station. It is then you may have prophetic dreams, ally dreams and warning dreams. I have learned so much about myself and the unconsciousness through dream work. I believe paying attention to dreams can be a direct line to increasing the gift of intuition.

Recently, I had this dream:

My cat is missing! She leaves the apartment without me knowing it. She is gone and I am so upset, berating myself for not paying attention and letting this happen. Then I thought (in the dream), "Where's George?" Oh no, my beloved little dog has disappeared, too! Why haven't I been more attentive about the apartment door being closed? How could I have let this happen?

The dream was telling me I would lose George by death the very next day (my cat, Momma Blue, had died months before). Both pets had "left the building."

Even if you get a premonition, there is often nothing you can do to change life. Although I hadn't interpreted my dream yet, I must have known something was going to happen because that day I spent some extra time with George, loving on him and giving him his favorite ear massage. At that time, I had no idea (consciously) it would be the last time I would look into those beautiful eyes—but maybe my intuition was giving me a dream to prepare my subconscious.

Most people have had these kinds of dreams, feelings and hunches, but they don't realize it is their intuition working for them. Pay attention and you may find you have a very helpful intuitive sense that you have never acknowledged.

You can begin to work with your intuition by making

that phone call to a friend when you begin thinking about her. Your hunch may be affirmed when she says, "Oh, I was just thinking about you!" Or "I just picked up the phone to call you and here you are calling me!" How did you know to make that call right then? That is your intuition!

To summarize:

- I believe that intuition is a soul level communication that can be nurtured by mindfulness, meditation, reflection, dream work and conscious acknowledgement. By listening to and acting on your "hunches," you can make them stronger. Intuition is like a muscle—as you exercise it, it will develop a strength that can be depended upon.

- Through time and experience, you will get to know your intuition by some sign or signs that you will learn to recognize: a shiver, a gut feeling, a change of mood, a heaviness or lightness in your body, or some sensation that is unique to you. Maybe you will hear a voice or an image will flash in your mind, you might get a "weird" feeling or you suddenly "lose" your thoughts and feel something instinctual.

- Intuition is your sixth sense and is as natural, useful and trustworthy as the five senses you are using already. Be grateful and acknowledge it, but don't talk too much about this inner gift you're cultivating, as many people are quick to judge something they don't understand. You don't need the negativity.

I hope I have given you a sense of what intuition is and the different ways you can access it. It's there just waiting to become a part of your life. Louise Hay says, "Your intuition knows what to do. The trick is getting your head to shut up so you can hear it."

Don't be afraid of it. Author Clarissa Estes Pinkola writes, "Intuition is the direct messenger of the soul." She encourages women to follow their instincts in her book, *Women Who Run with the Wolves.* Speaking of books, I have developed the talent of being able to find information and messages through books. I ask the question and then pull out a book and open it to a random page. It is uncanny, what I read always seems to address my question in some way! I intend to continue to recognize this growing ability.

Be curious regarding how soul messages will manifest for you: a voice, a shiver, a dream, a song that keeps going around and around in your head. As always, my advice is to pay attention to everything! Yesterday, I noticed the Thomas' English Muffins package was imprinted with "Wake up to what's possible" on the plastic wrap. *Okay,* I said to myself, *I will!* There are all kinds of possibilities out there for us to see with fresh eyes.

"It is always with excitement that I wake up in the morning wondering what my intuition will toss up to me, like gifts from the sea. I work with it and rely on it. It is my partner," says Dr. Jonas Salk.

And so, I begin my day, looking for clues and guidance

for all the possibilities that my life presents to me. I am inspired by a teacher in my life, the incredible Edgar Cayce, the Sleeping Prophet, who said in one of his readings given while in a trance, "The more and more each is inspired by that which is intuitive or the relying upon the soul force within, the greater, the farther, the deeper, the broader, the more constructive may be the result."

In her book, *Women's Bodies, Women's Wisdom*, Dr. Christiane Northrup addresses intuition by saying, "Our inner guidance comes to us first through our feeling and body wisdom—not through intellectual understanding." She continues to say, "Intuition is a natural way of knowing which often gets shut down around the age of seven."

Our technological culture teaches us to value our rational, logical thinking and dismiss other ways of knowing. Northrup believes that by becoming more inwardly directed, we will have access to our intuition, saying, "God is within every one of us and speaks through inner guidance."

So, go for it! Pay attention to the guidance you will find everywhere, even on the back of a dump truck or a slogan on the wrapper of English muffins. Look for that sign or symbol, listen to that inner or outer voice, value that impulse or emotion, connect that inner nudge to your daily decisions and honor your soul force.

Albert Einstein said, "The intuitive mind is a sacred gift and the rational mind is a faithful servant. We have created a society that honors the servant and has forgotten the gift."

CHAPTER 25

A "Whole Brain" Approach to Making Decisions

What shall I do? Who can I trust? Can I trust myself in making this decision?

Decisions regarding a life-threatening illness can be confusing, overwhelming and even tormenting. Here are some pointers on how to make educated decisions based on information, research and logic (from the left brain), balanced with intuition and inner guidance (from your right brain).

Begin with your doctor's assessment of your situation. Perfect health may be an unreasonable goal, so ask your doctor what are realistic goals? (See Chapter Twenty-six: Questions to Ask Your Doctor.) I recommend writing everything down because often the brain short-circuits when we are stressed and valuable information can slip away as soon as you walk out of the doctor's office.

Make sure you have all the vital information from your doctor and everything is spelled correctly: the diagnosis, procedures and drugs. It's a great help, too, if you have someone who will go to the doctor's appointments with you and take notes.

The best decisions can be made when using both sides of the brain. Therefore, you will see the two columns I have created that are calculated to engage both sides of the brain. The process of working with these questions will give you two types of information in order to help you make a balanced, *whole brain* decision.

Write down the situation or the decision you are considering and include the date at the top of your paper. Next, read through the following lists and choose one exercise from each side. They do not have to correlate in any way, just make sure you do some from both lists. Don't labor too long on each topic; quickly write down whatever thoughts occur to you. There is no particular order in which to do them. And you can do them more than once.

Left Brain	**Right Brain**
Gather facts.	How do you feel about the facts?
Do research on your own.	Are you asking the right questions?
Get feedback from doctors.	Get feedback from your body.
What are you thinking?	What is your intuition saying?
Get a second opinion.	Imagine a favorable outcome.

Review and update notes.

What are your doctor's credentials?

Compare pain versus gain.

List the pros and cons of the decision.

What kind of support/ therapy is available?

Make sure you have all your questions answered.

Write out the time-line and check it with your doctor.

Write affirmations of positive outcomes.

Pinpoint your confusion.

Does the diagnosis make sense?

Talk to someone who has made a similar decision.

Evaluate your doctor's skills and history.

Investigate the hospital your doctor uses.

Is there anything that doesn't feel right?

Explore other medical options.

Draw a doodle—an abstract picture of pain.

Mull over options in a hypnagogic state.

Ask your best friend for advice and feedback.

Write or reflect on your feelings.

Design a healing image.

Meditate on the affirmations.

Write or draw about the confusion.

What is your "gut" telling you?

Confide your fears in someone.

Do you trust your doctors?

Listen to uplifting music.

What kind of extra support do you need?	Do you need spiritual counseling?
Read an inspiring book.	Reflect on your life.
Talk over any frustration with your doctors.	Draw your anger.
Research alternative treatments.	Contemplate surrender and acceptance.
Pray. (Talk to God.)	Meditate. (Listen to God.)

Write down any other questions or thoughts as they occur to you. Approach this *whole brain* exercise with no judgements. Let your intuition decide what to work on and in what order. You can create a folder with your drawings, writing and notes. You may want to keep it private or share it with a trusted loved one. You will feel more in control when you do the exercises and they will help you make the best decisions for you.

The information on the two hemispheres of the brain and how they function has been around since the 1980's. I learned about it from a book called, *Drawing on the Right Side of the Brain,* by Dr. Betty Edwards. For over 30 years, I taught hundreds of people how to draw using techniques to access their right hemispheres. Much to their surprise, they picked up on the idea quickly—shifting into a way that an artist sees. This shift is achieved through unusual exercises which take the reader out of their habitual ways of thinking. Edwards' book is full of fun art exercises to help you shift into the right hemisphere. Dr. Betty

Edwards has also written another amazing book called, *Drawing on the Artist Within*, in which she shows you how to use symbols to help you solve problems.

We live in a technological, linear society where words dominate. We are taught to think sequentially and put the puzzle together piece by piece. We need to balance this way of thinking with images, music, poetry, emotions, art, spirituality—for then can we become a whole brain person who can use both sides of the brain to handle life's situations.

Most of us get stuck in our favored or habitual hemisphere because it is just more comfortable there. To ask yourself while you are in a right brain mode to pay bills or make those necessary phone calls is like pulling teeth. The smart thing to do is to assess the situation and decide which side of the brain you need to be in for the best results.

You can change your posture or body position as a simple way to switch over. Sit up straight in a chair at a desk with no distractions when you are doing bookkeeping or taking a test for instance. Stretch out and lounge on the couch if you are imagining taking a trip or contemplating a new creative project.

Predominantly left-brained people will thrive on doing things in a linear, sequential, logical way but feel uncomfortable doing something that is completely without directions. Predominantly right-brained people will love to "wing it," let creativity flow and then make something original if they mess up! Both sides have their talents and strengths. It helps to know which side of your brain you favor and be able to choose the side that is best for the task at hand.

Rarely is there only one way to approach a task. For example, painting a picture may involve left brain choices such as preparing the canvas, choosing the right tools, doing some research on the subject and making sure you are in paint clothes. Then the right brain needs to take over to get creative. There is the evaluating and analyzing that the left brain likes to do at different stages of completion. Should that color be redder or more orange? What about the composition, should it be more dynamic? How would I do that? The right brain might want to view it from across the room for a fresh perspective or turn it upside down and see what it looks like that way. The left brain might evaluate the technique and look for any errors in perspective while the right brain is more interested in the emotional impact of the design and colors. The left brain can then make judgements on how to frame the artwork. Back and forth the brain works, judging and expressing, correcting and intuiting. For most of us, this process is very fluid.

The exercises I developed at the beginning of the chapter are designed to address both sides of the brain in order to make sure you have covered all your bases when making a decision. You can learn to use both sides of your brain and not be a half-wit!

CHAPTER 26

Questions to Ask Your Doctor

When we, as patients, enter a doctor's office, we often go into a stress-induced brain fog and forget all those details and questions we want addressed. To help you stay focused, here is a list of questions for you to ask your doctor. Take what is applicable to your situation and be prepared to take notes.

What is the name of my condition? (Make sure to have the correct spelling.)

What is the proposed treatment plan?

How costly is the treatment or surgery and will my insurance pay for it?

How long will the treatment last?

What is the time-line?

What do statistics say about outcomes?

What are the risks?

What are the side-effects?

What can I do now to prepare for treatment?

Where can I find more information?

What are the long-term effects?

What about expected pain levels?

What are options for pain control?

Will I have scars?

Will any physical therapy be needed?

Will I need blood transfusions?

Can I give my blood in advance?

Will I need a nurse or home caregiver at any stage of the treatment?

What will my physical limitations be in the future?

Are there mental health professionals available if needed? (Through the hospital system)

Is there a spiritual counselor available if I want one? (Many hospitals have one on staff)

Who can I call with questions? Will someone reply to emails and phone messages?

How will my diet or life-style activities be affected?

What are the next options if this process or surgery isn't successful?

What does recovery look like?

What is the goal of my treatment?

Are there any advantages of genetic testing?

Should I consider any clinical trials?

Can you recommend any studies or articles to read?

Why are you recommending this treatment at this particular time?

What is your experience with this treatment?

What kind of anesthesia will be used?

How long will I be in the hospital?

How many times have you (the doctor and/or surgeon) performed this surgery or procedure?

Who will be assisting you? Will I meet them before the surgery?

What influences your choices? What are your past experiences?

Will I be re-evaluated or tested before surgery to see if anything has changed?

What can my loved ones expect?

Do you have a copy of my DNR order? Power of Attorney?

How do I conduct my daily life, work life, sex life and exercise, now and after treatment?

If I refuse your treatment plan, can I remain your patient?

Do you have all the information you need regarding my medical history?

Are you aware of my allergies and current medications?

Are there any vitamins, supplements, foods or herbal products that are contra-indicated?

Do you have a list of the medicines I am taking? Any that I should stop taking or change?

Be sure to ask anything that concerns you. You have a right to ask whatever you want and your doctor or staff should respond or get back to you with answers. Always take notes and date them. I emphasize this over and over because you may not remember everything when you are stressed. It is helpful to have another person by your side for support, to take notes and to make sure your questions get answered. If your doctor is evasive, annoyed, vague, dismissive or too busy to address your concerns and questions, you may want to change doctors.

Go through the questions listed and choose the ones you want to ask. If you have many, give your doctor a list of them and ask for the answers in a reasonable amount of time. If the doctor is too busy to call, there is always the nurse or a staff person who can call, fax or email you the answers. Be thorough, be persistent and be discerning; it's your life we are talking about!

CHAPTER 27

Recommended Books

The Picture of Health: Healing Your Life with Art, by Lucia Capacchione, shares how she healed her illness by originating right brain art exercises. Through these, she helps the reader access the inner healer, inner wise counselor and inner child through a simple process anyone can do. She has also written two other books I recommend: *The Power of the Other Hand* and *The Creative Journal. The Power of the Other Hand* is a book about channeling the inner wisdom of the right brain by using your non-dominant hand (for most of us it is the left hand). This technique connects you to a completely different part of the brain where you can access your inner child, your spiritual self and the healer within. Through simple exercises using pen and paper, you can have a conversation with both sides of your brain using your right and left hands. I find the exercises powerful, inspiring and helpful.

Drawing on the Right Side of the Brain and *Drawing on the Artist Within* are two books written by Dr. Betty Edwards.

They are filled with research regarding the brain, exercises on how to use the right brain for art and creative thinking, and they are illustrated with many examples of drawing techniques and problem solving. Anyone can be an artist once they engage the right side of the brain!

Writing Down Your Soul and *The Lotus and the Lily*, by Janet Conner, are two unique books for those who resonate with reflective inspiring writing exercises and spiritual direction. The author tells how she saved her own life through reflection and forgiveness, and she presents good information on how we can follow her lead.

Zen Mind, Beginner's Mind, by Shunryu Suzuki, is a classic book on the practice and philosophy of Zen, written simply and beautifully to the point.

A Course in Miracles is a channeled book that appeared in the 1970's and took the world by storm. This is a book you will love and resist—with new ideas that will turn your world upside down. Try not to throw it across the room, as many people have done in their frustration, as they attempt to follow the material presented.

The Power of Now and *A New Earth* are two classics by Eckhart Tolle. Tolle is a contemporary author who had a mystical experience after years of depression. His writing, so wise and clear, is meant to wake us up to our highest purpose. His workshops and talks, available on CD, are enhanced by his fey sense of humor. Giggle along with him as he shares his brilliant insights.

You are the Placebo, Evolve Your Brain, Breaking the Habit of Being Yourself, and *Becoming Supernatural* are four wonderful books about how meditation changes the brain—and how the latest research in neuroscience proves it. Author Joe Dispenza has included the proof with photos of brain images from people in his workshops. He also has several wonderful guided meditations at the end of the book: *You are the Placebo.*

Close to the Bone: *Life-Threatening Illness as a Soul Journey,* by Jean Shinoda Bolen, is a deeply satisfying book on life-changing illnesses recorded from ancient history, mythology, and her years of being a therapist, including her journey with the long-term illness and death of her young adult son.

Loving What Is (and any book by Byron Katie) is filled with simple techniques which provide a startling short-cut to being honest with yourself and your life. She is known for "The Work" which consists of four questions of inquiry that bring you to terms with reality. The chapter called *Making Friends with the Worst That Can Happen* in this book is very helpful if you are considering death as an impending possibility.

Dream Work: Techniques for Discovering the Creative Power in Dreams and *Where People Fly and Water Runs Uphill* are two great books written by one of the founding fathers of current dream study. Reverend Jeremy Taylor, whose "take" on the importance of studying our dreams is so inspiring, you will want to start dream work immediately!

The Healing Power of Dreams: Techniques for Interpreting and Using Your Dreams to Reveal Hidden Health Problems, Speed Your Recovery, and Promote Lifelong Health, is by Patricia Garfield, one of the founding mothers of dream study. Her personal story of healing is intertwined in this book which makes it all the more interesting.

The Secret Language of Your Body: The Essential Guide to Health and Wellness, by Inna Segal, is a guide for the emotional, mental and energetic causes of disease and presents ten basic principles of healing. Her material is broken down into categories of the different parts of the body and how they correlate with symptoms.

The Healing Power of Illness: The Meaning of Symptoms and How to Interpret Them by Thorwald Dethlefsen and Rudiger Dahlke, M.D., is one of the most helpful books I've read on the connection between the body and mind. The authors present the bold and uncomfortable argument that the patient is "not the innocent victim of his or her own sickness." The book delves into the meanings of symptoms and the "why" of disease.

Cell-Level Healing: The Bridge from Soul to Cell, by Joyce Whiteley Hawkes, Ph.D., is the story of how a scientist became a healer after a blow to her head knocked her into an out-of-body experience. Her photos and information about cells are incredible, as are her many healing meditation scripts.

Bone: Dying into Life, by Marion Woodman, is written from the journal she kept during her experience of living with cancer of the uterus. Woodman used her knowledge of the archetypal forces interacting in her illness to help heal herself. She presents psychological information as only a Jungian analyst can do. Woodman's story will be of interest to those who are open to the influence of the unconscious.

Learning to Breathe, by Priscilla Warner, references a year long quest she undertook to bring calm into her life and to heal the panic attacks that left her fighting for her breath. The reader will be taken on an exploration of many modalities she tried including a mystical rabbi, a Buddhist meditation teacher, and a variety of therapists, healers and neuroscientists. Her search for a cure is full of surprises.

The Master Speaks and *Realization of Oneness,* by Joel Goldsmith, are two of my favorites from my library of Goldsmith books. I think these books are a precursor to *A Course in Miracles.* Goldsmith's writings have a Biblical flavor and patriarchal language that may turn some off, but if you can get over that, his writing is a goldmine for seekers.

Never Fear Cancer Again: How to Prevent and Reverse Cancer, by Raymond Francis, M.Sc., is about how he helped his brother heal his cancer. The six pathways he addresses are: nutrition, toxins, mental, physical, genetic and medical. He talks about supplements and lists the amounts needed. According to him, there are only two causes of disease—biochemical deficiency and toxins.

Cellular Health Series: Cancer by Matthias Rath, M. D. is a little booklet that packs in lots of information about the importance of collagen, lysine and vitamin C. Locate his booklet through his website: www.drrathresearch.org. He believes that disease originates inside a vulnerable cell and bio-energetic carriers such as collagen are the key to a healthy cell.

The Alchemy of Illness by Kat Duff is one of my favorite books. I've read it twice and often find myself dipping into it, enjoying her nuggets of wisdom on every page. I love what she reveals about shame, writing in such a novel way about its gifts. She writes from her experience of years of suffering with Chronic Fatigue Immune Deficiency Syndrome.

Your Body Doesn't Lie: Unlock the Power of Your Natural Energy and *Life Energy: Using the Meridians to Unlock the Hidden Power of Your Emotions* are two classics by Dr. John Diamond who draws from the kinesiology work of Dr. George Goodheart. Dr. Diamond shows how to determine the level of your life energy and discover what emotional factors are interfering with your health's expression. The books provide directions on how to use a simple muscle test to let your body diagnose the problem. This technique works well for some and not so well for others. Also, there are good instructions for strengthening the thymus and using positive affirmations as part of the healing process.

Healing Dreams: Exploring the Dreams That Can Transform Your Life, by Marc Ian Barasch, covers an amazing scope of dream work with examples of dreams from all over the world. Also covered are healing dreams and the questions they ask of us, healing the shadow, spiritual dreams, individual stories and much more. Barasch is a brilliant writer and includes many inspiring stories. This is a must-read and has become a classic and a favorite of mine to dip into for words of wisdom. *The Healing Path: A Soul Approach to Illness*, also by Marc Ian Barasch, presents an answer to what disease is and how can we handle the contradictions it presents. It includes the author's fascinating worldwide search to heal his own disease— cancer of the thyroid.

Sidewalk Oracles: Playing with Signs, Symbols and Synchronicity in Everyday Life, by Robert Moss, offers a way to "carry your dream in your pocket" as you go throughout your day. Observe what symbols appear around you from everywhere including the sidewalk as you stroll along. Moss has several unusual books out, including *Dreamways of the Iroquois: Honoring the Secret Wishes of the Soul*, about his dreams and encounters with Iroquois wisdom keepers. He also gives directions for his lightning fast approach to working with dreams.

Inner Work: Using Dreams and Active Imagination for Personal Growth, by Robert Johnson, gives direct approaches to analyzing your dreams and working with symbols using active imagination and a four-step process.

The Woman's Dictionary of Symbols and Sacred Objects, by Barbara Walker, is a comprehensive look at symbols around the world and through herstory. It is an impressive encyclopedia with many illustrations. It is an excellent reference book to have in your library.

Dreams and Guided Imagery: Gifts for Transforming Illness and Crisis, by Tallulah Lyons, is a unique book that is written in such a way that takes the reader into the midst of dream group dynamics. Her book also includes scripts for the reader to use to work with the images and symbols that appear to them. She worked for fifteen years in hospital locations facilitating dream circles with cancer patients. Read more in my interview with Tallulah in the chapter on dreams.

The Divided Mind, by Dr. John Sarno, is written by a medical doctor and professor who has also written *Healing Back Pain.* Both books address the mind-body connection. He traces the beginnings of psychosomatic illness, it's nature and how to work with the mind to heal illnesses. Dr. Sarno believes we are internally at war—thus the title, *The Divided Mind.* He believes the dynamics involved in pain, when once understood, can allow for healing to occur.

The Four Agreements, by Don Miguel Ruiz, is a short book with a simple message that our beliefs often rob us of joy and take us off the path of enlightenment. The Four Agreements originate from Toltec wisdom coming from ancient Mexican mystics called "naguals." The introduction and first chapter are mind-blowing regarding the dream of what we call reality.

kathleenmillat42@gmail.com. Contact the author for permission to quote or reproduce any material in the *Year of the Onion.*

Acknowledgements

I want to thank my editor (and daughter) Shanen Johnson for helping me birth this book. It's a little book not weighing quite a pound, but it took a lot of big pushes to get it out into the world! I'm so grateful you were there on my cancer journey supporting me and loving me through it. I never dreamed you would be so strong. I am one lucky mother.

Much gratitude goes to my doctors (whose names in my book were "doctored") for their skills, kindness and dedication, to the nurses who were so competent and caring and to all the wonderful staff at Medical University of South Carolina (MUSC), Hollings Cancer Center and Mayo Clinic.

To my family and friends—your support kept me afloat on this adventure of a lifetime.

I acknowledge myself for staying sane while dealing with cancer. I learned new talents of whistling in the dark and balancing on a tight-rope. Writing this book was the final piece of my journey. I present it to the world with the wish that it will help those individuals who need it.

I want to remember my loved ones who died in 2019: my sweetheart, Nick and my funny cat, Momma Blue. And then in September 2020, our precious dog, George died unexpectedly. You three will always be part of my life. You are gone, but not forgotten.

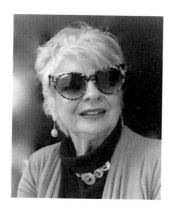

ABOUT THE AUTHOR

Kathleen Millat Johnson is a writer and artist living in Summerville, South Carolina. Originally from Dayton, Ohio, Kathleen discovered the beauty of the Lowcountry when she moved to the South in 1999.

Kathleen has enjoyed a career in art and teaching, written for newspapers and magazines, created and produced a play and documentary film, and originated events that celebrate women and their talents.

Kathleen's life has been enriched and guided through her study of dreams and symbols. She enjoys sharing these ideas and practices through workshops and consultations. Other interests include being an advocate for women, fundraising for education and working for animal welfare.

She lives with her grandson, Jonathan, and daughter, Shanen Johnson, who was the editor, photographer and cover designer for the *Year of the Onion: A Healing Journey with Cancer*.

Notes

Notes

Notes

Notes

Notes

Notes

Notes

Notes